Doctors and
Their Workshops

A National Bureau
of Economic Research
Monograph

Doctors and Their Workshops: Economic Models of Physician Behavior

Mark V. Pauly

The University of Chicago Press

Chicago and London

Mark V. Pauly is professor of economics at
Northwestern University.

The University of Chicago Press, Chicago 60637
The University of Chicago Press, Ltd., London

© 1980 by the University of Chicago
All rights reserved. Published 1980
Printed in the United States of America
84 83 82 81 80   5 4 3 2 1

Library of Congress Cataloging in Publication Data

Pauly, Mark V   1941–
  Doctors and their workshops.

  (A National Bureau of Economic Research monograph)
  Includes bibliographical references and index.
  1. Medical economics—United States. 2. Physicians—
United States. 3. Medical care—United States—
Utilization. 4. Physician and patient—United States.
I. Title. II. Series: National Bureau of
Economic Research. National Bureau of Economic
Research monograph.
RA410.53.P36   338.4'56136210973   80–16112
ISBN 0–226–65044–8

Contents

Contents

Relation of the Directors to the
Work and Publications of the
National Bureau of Economic Research

1. The object of the National Bureau of Economic Research is to ascertain and to present to the public important economic facts and their interpretation in a scientific and impartial manner. The Board of Directors is charged with the responsibility of ensuring that the work of the National Bureau is carried on in strict conformity with this object.

2. The President of the National Bureau shall submit to the Board of Directors, or to its Executive Committee, for their formal adoption all specific proposals for research to be instituted.

3. No research report shall be published by the National Bureau until the President has sent each member of the Board a notice that a manuscript is recommended for publication and that in the President's opinion it is suitable for publication in accordance with the principles of the National Bureau. Such notification will include an abstract or summary of the manuscript's content and a response form for use by those Directors who desire a copy of the manuscript for review. Each manuscript shall contain a summary drawing attention to the nature and treatment of the problem studied, the character of the data and their utilization in the report, and the main conclusions reached.

4. For each manuscript so submitted, a special committee of the Directors (including Directors Emeriti) shall be appointed by majority agreement of the President and Vice Presidents (or by the Executive Committee in case of inability to decide on the part of the President and Vice Presidents), consisting of three Directors selected as nearly as may be one from each general division of the Board. The names of the special manuscript committee shall be stated to each Director when notice of the proposed publication is submitted to him. It shall be the duty of each member of the special manuscript committee to read the manuscript. If each member of the manuscript committee signifies his approval within thirty days of the transmittal of the manuscript, the report may be published. If at the end of that period any member of the manuscript committee withholds his approval, the President shall then notify each member of the Board, requesting approval or disapproval of publication, and thirty days additional shall be granted for this purpose. The manuscript shall then not be published unless at least a majority of the entire Board who shall have voted on the proposal within the time fixed for the receipt of votes shall have approved.

5. No manuscript may be published, though approved by each member of the special manuscript committee, until forty-five days have elapsed from the transmittal of the report in manuscript form. The interval is allowed for the receipt of any memorandum of dissent or reservation, together with a brief statement of his reasons, that any member may wish to express; and such memorandum of dissent or reservation shall be published with the manuscript if he so desires. Publication does not, however, imply that each member of the Board has read the manuscript, or that either members of the Board in general or the special committee have passed on its validity in every detail.

6. Publications of the National Bureau issued for informational purposes concerning the work of the Bureau and its staff, or issued to inform the public of activities of Bureau staff, and volumes issued as a result of various conferences involving the National Bureau shall contain a specific disclaimer noting that such publication has not passed through the normal review procedures required in this resolution. The Executive Committee of the Board is charged with review of all such publications from time to time to ensure that they do not take on the character of formal research reports of the National Bureau, requiring formal Board approval.

7. Unless otherwise determined by the Board or exempted by the terms of paragraph 6, a copy of this resolution shall be printed in each National Bureau publication.

(Resolution adopted October 25, 1926, as revised through September 30, 1974)

Acknowledgments

This book summarizes research begun when I was a faculty research fellow at the Center for Economic Analysis of Human Behavior and Social Institutions, National Bureau of Economic Research, Palo Alto, during the academic year 1974–75. Victor Fuchs encouraged me to start and to pursue these topics, and his criticisms and comments were most helpful during the course of the research and writing. I also received helpful comments and advice (though not necessarily agreement with conclusions) from Robert Evans, Barry Friedman, Gerry Goldstein, William Gould, Jerry Green, Michael Grossman, Joseph Newhouse, and Richard Rosett. Jan Platt helped me get started with the empirical work, and special thanks are due to Tryfon Beazoglou for exceptional research assistance.

M. P.

1   Physicians as Agents

Total medical care expenditures in the United States in 1978 were $192 billion. Of that amount, $35.3 billion, or only 18.3%, represented payments for physicians' services. In the manufacturing sector, profits before taxes were about 13% of total expenditures. Looking at this first set of figures, one might be tempted to conclude that physicians are of relatively minor importance in the health care system, and that the prices, fees, or other incentives which they experience are of little consequence. In a sense this is true; a substantial reduction in physician fees (say, 25%) would have little effect on total medical spending.[1] By the same token, however, a 25% reduction in profits would have little effect on most product prices. The major theme of this study is that physician-returns play a role in the medical care sector which is analogous to that played by profits in the for-profit sector. Just as the incentive provided by the relatively small fraction of total spending that is profits determines the form and use of all inputs and outputs in conventional markets, similarly the relatively small amount that goes to physicians provides the financial incentive which determines the bulk of resource use, output quantities and characteristics, and total costs in the health sector.

There has been fairly extensive study of the market for physicians' services, and of physician time as an input into these services, especially with regard to physician provision of ambulatory care. The general focus of the analysis here is different: this analysis will be concerned with the effects physicians have on the use of medical inputs other than the physician's own input or those inputs for which he pays directly. There will be a similar consideration of the effects of physicians and physician incentives on the markets for kinds of medical care other than physician's services. Physician behavior will be examined not just in the office, but also in the hospital and in all of the physician's "workshops." The

1

focus will be not just on the physician's own actions, but also on the effects of those actions on the environment in which he works and on the resources with which he works.

The parallel which has been drawn between physician expenditures and profits, like all analogies, is not perfect. There are some additional aspects of physician behavior to be emphasized. The most important of these is the physician's role as provider of information to demanders. The physician not only coordinates the output production process, as does the classical entrepreneur, but he also provides information to potential demanders on the need for and value of services that he or others will provide. This represents a kind of relationship between buyer and seller which falls outside the scope of the standard neoclassical models, whether competitive or monopolistic. While there are some similarities between physician advice and advertising, the integration of information and services provision will be the most distinctive feature of the models that will be discussed.

A second difference concerns what might be reasonable to postulate as the physician's maximand. Maximizing profits is an acceptable assumption for most businesses, but maximization solely of physician money income is not a plausible assumption for physicians. Instead, much of what is to be explained empirically will require broadening the set of arguments that concern the physician's utility function. While models of a utility-maximizing entrepreneur are not unknown, the economy of theory and the empirical relevance of the money income maximization approach will not be available in this study.

The physician, like the classical entrepreneur, really performs two functions: (1) he organizes and directs the production process, and (2) he provides some productive input. In the case of the entrepreneur, his equity capital investment provides some of the firm's capital stock. In the case of the physician, his own time is a useful and often essential productive unit. While the importance of capital to the production of output has always been recognized, and while the role of physician time in the production of office-based ambulatory care has also been subject to scrutiny, an important part of total physician time has been ignored or treated haphazardly. This is the time the physician spends caring for patients in hospitals. The fraction of total working time spent at the hospital varies according to the physician's specialization, of course, but what sketchy information we have suggests that it averages about 30% of physician time, and may be more than half of total time for the hospital-oriented surgical specialties.[2] In order to round out our understanding of how physicians affect the use of all inputs, including those not paid for by the physician, it is necessary to incorporate physicians' time into the analysis of hospital production.

In principle, of course, physician time input also affects the productivity of other ways of treating patients. More time spent diagnosing or monitoring may make drug therapy more effective and nursing home care more productive. But it will not be possible to treat those subjects here.

A Taxonomy of Physician Pricing Models

In order to explain how physicians affect the use of other inputs, we need to understand how physician prices are set. This is ultimately an empirical question, on which there is presently no consensus. It will be helpful to try to classify alternative theories which have been suggested. Figure 1, an extension of a scheme developed by Uwe Reinhardt,[3] provides one such classification.

Market situation / Physician Pricing	Market clears, demand not shifted	Market doesn't clear; demand not shifted	Market clears; demand shifted
Price-taker	1 Competitive equilibrium	3 Price ceiling	5 Oligopolistic demand creation; target income
Price-setter	2 Monopoly equilibrium	4 Chronic excess demand	6 Shift of entire demand curve

The rows refer to the extent of individual physician control over price. The physician may, as in the first row, take a going price as given, either because competition forces him to do so, or because insurance reimbursement policy, administrative difficulties of changing prices, or government price controls compel him to accept a given price for any output he produces. In the other row, the physician is assumed to have some control over the price he can charge and still obtain business. The columns reflect alternative assumptions, one dealing with whether or not the price attains a level at which supply and demand are equated, and the market clears; the other dealing with whether or not the individual physician is able to shift the demand for his own services by varying what he suggests to patients. (There could also be a fourth column, in which demand is shifted and markets do not clear, but that would only represent a combination of the second and third columns.)

The cells provide a way to classify possible models. Cell 1 would be the usual competitive market. If the physician services' market were of this nature, both demand and supply curves could be estimated. If the market were the standard textbook monopoly in cell 2, the market, individual, or firm-level demand curves could be estimated. It would not, however, be possible to estimate a firm or physician supply curve of output. The output the monopolist physician would choose would depend upon the configuration of the entire demand curve, not just the price he happened to charge. There are some assumptions that might be made which would make it possible to estimate a quasi-supply curve or offer curve, but it is not clear that these assumptions would be legitimate.

So far, however, these are standard problems in estimating models of any market. The peculiar problems of the medical care industry begin to emerge in the other cells. A price which physicians take as given may be set below the level which permits markets to clear, as in cell 3. This is most likely to happen if, either because of insurance reimbursement limits or because of price controls, the price is not permitted to rise. It may also represent a state of disequilibrium, in which prices are gradually rising to their equilibrium levels. In this case, no demand curve for physician services can be estimated; the only points observed are those on the supply curve.

In cell 4 the physician controls his own price. If he is an income maximizer, he would set the price at the monopoly level, and satisfy all the demand at that price. But he may have goals other than income, and pursuit of these goals may prompt him to set price below the monopoly level, and refuse to produce enough to satisfy the demand at that price.

The distinction between cells 3 and 4 arises from the source of excess demand. In cell 3, price is exogenous to any individual physician. In such a case, it is the constraint on his willingness to supply that causes excess demand to occur. Excess demand may arise for the usual reason: price may equal the physician's marginal cost (including the opportunity cost of his own time) at a quantity which is less than that demanded from him. If he has preferences as to the kinds of cases he will treat, it is possible to have excess demand for some kinds, while other, more desirable kinds are selected to be treated. The trade-off between leisure and work may depend on the kind of work to be done. If there is an "insufficient" amount of desirable cases, he may not be willing to supply as much labor time at a given price as when the mix of outputs is more to his liking.

In cell 4, however, the physician sets the price. He may not be willing to produce all of the output demanded at this price, for the reasons to be discussed later. In this case we obviously cannot observe the demand curve. It is also true that we cannot observe a supply curve either, since the monopolist by definition is not able to sell all he wants at given prices. In cell 3 excess demand need not require physicians to have more in their utility functions than income and leisure, if prices are fixed by law or are sticky. But in cell 4 excess demand can only exist if physicians for some reason receive utility from its existence.

In all of these cases, the individual physician takes the demand curve which confronts him as given. We will now consider models in which the physician can create or shift the demand curve which confronts him. In cell 5, he would obviously only have an incentive to do so if price exceeds marginal opportunity cost; at prices below that point, the situation is the same as that in cell 3. If price is above marginal cost, it is possible to show how demand will be created (this will be done in a later chapter).

Finally, in cell 6 the physician chooses the price he wishes to charge on a demand curve which he manipulates. Precise analysis is difficult here because behavior depends on the way in which the demand curve shifts as information is changed, and there are no comfortable a priori conjectures on this. We can, however, use this model to provide some conditional statements about market response.

The Physician as Agent

Many medical goods and services are not demanded directly by patients, but are requested on the patient's behalf by a physician. Indeed, in some cases, such as prescription drugs or hospital care, the patient is not even legally permitted to demand the items. And yet economists have persisted in estimating consumer demand curves for medical care in the same way as for other goods over whose purchase the consumer has direct control. How can the supposed response of use to consumer income and user price be rationalized when consumers are not, in large part, making the relevant decisions? Feldstein has suggested that an answer might be constructed on an assumption that the physician acts as the patient's agent.[4] In this role, the physician demands (or has the patient acquiesce in demanding) exactly those quantities of care of various types that the patient would choose if he had the information and knowledge that the physician has.[5] If the physician were to act as a pure or perfect agent, his ostensible maximand would be the patient's utility, and his choices would duplicate the choices the patient would make, if the patient had the same information as does the physician.

While much of medical ethics can be interpreted as an attempt to use moral suasion to persuade physicians to adopt the agent's role, there are reasons to expect that the physician may not act as a pure agent and that his maximand need not be the fully informed patient's maximand. First, it is not obvious that any physician will have the information needed to permit him to act as a perfect agent, even if he wishes to do so. While the patient may be ignorant about the way to produce health or other attributes of medical care, he alone knows how much health he desires. The physician may be better informed about the technology for producing health, but he may be poorly informed about the patient's demand for health. On balance, the patient may be better informed than the physician. This assymetry of information has often been noted, but it has less often been recognized that it is an assymetry in type of information, not necessarily in amount. Indeed, Smallwood and Smith have even suggested that, when confronted with the difficult task of reading his patient's preferences, the physician may give up altogether and concentrate only on equal physically measurable outputs, such as changes in probability of death.[6] Whether or not physicians behave in this way, it is worth noting that physician ignorance can be as important as patient ignorance in causing deviations of actual from ideal outcomes.[7]

Second, even if he had the requisite information, the physician may not in fact act as a perfect agent. It is not usually assumed that any other economic actor chooses only with the interests of his customer in mind. From Adam Smith on, economists have argued that benevolence in producers of goods and services is neither to be expected nor necessarily desired. But if the physician manages the care of the patient with his own interests—income, leisure, interest of work—in mind, then he would not necessarily be acting as a perfect agent.

Thus there are reasons to expect that the agency relationship will not be perfect. But in order to get much further, two additional questions must be answered. How would the physician be expected to act if he is *not* acting as the patient's agent? And equally important, how is the extent of his departure from perfect agency determined? I intend to show that it will generally be both possible and likely that the physician will depart from the role of perfect agent, but that there are constraints on the extent of this departure. Perhaps more surprisingly, I shall show that the physician will choose medical care inputs so as to minimize the cost of producing a given level of health *even if he is not acting as the patient's agent, but rather as a selfish income maximizer.* I shall show that, given a suitably broad definition of cost, a similar proposition holds for a much wider class of physician utility functions as well.

Some Difficulties in the Notion of Agency

The concept of agency is most transparent for the situation in which all services are sold in competitive markets. The agent's only task then is to choose the quantities of those inputs that would be demanded by the consumer at the given prices if the consumer had as much information as the agent has. That one of the services may be produced by the agent is of little consequence. As long as the agent accepts the price as given, and believes that he can sell as much as he wishes at that price, the agent has no incentive to alter the quantity of any service that any individual consumer demands, and no ability to alter the price he pays. Of course, if consumers are so poorly informed as to need agents, then a competitive market might not emerge. However, if some consumers are well informed, even if others are not, a competitive market may exist, and agents may behave optimally.

When the agent is also a monopolist in the provision of some productive input, there are two possible assumptions one might make. One might assume that he has the patient demand the quantities a fully informed patient would demand if price were set equal to marginal cost. Alternatively, the agent might try to determine the quantity that patients would demand at any given price if they were informed. Then, given this "true" demand curve, the physician would set the price at the monopoly level, and recommend the "fully informed" quantity corresponding to that price.

If the market is perfectly competitive, there is no reason for the physician not to act as a pure agent, while if the market is monopolistic, it appears to be inconsistent to assume that the physician is an income maximizer when he sets prices but not when he offers advice. The same motivation which leads him to set prices above marginal cost will lead him to distort the advice he gives.

A second difficulty with the agency notion arises in situations in which the quantity used is not the quantity that would be demanded by fully informed consumers when price equals social marginal cost. One possibility is that there is excess demand. If the physician were to act as the agent for a given patient, he would choose to satisfy that patient's fully informed demand. But if supply constraints make it impossible for him to do so for all patients, then the physician cannot feasibly act as a perfect agent for all patients.

A somewhat similar problem arises when insurance covers all or part of the cost of services the physician orders. From the viewpoint of any individual patient, his utility is maximized if he receives (approximately) the quantity he would have demanded if he were fully informed and faced a price equal to the net or user price. Even though the value to him of the last units he purchases is probably less than their social marginal cost, he ignores this "welfare loss" because the cost is spread over the usually very numerous other insureds. Even an individual physician's entire list of patients is likely to be a sufficiently small fraction of total insureds to permit the physician to ignore this welfare loss. But consumers would prefer that all physicians adopt a rationing policy in which they receive the quantity they would have demanded at price equalling marginal cost, not the quantity at which price equals the marginal user price. However, one would not expect the individual physicians to adopt such a rationing policy. When insurance is present, we need to recognize that it may not maximize aggregate patient welfare if each physician acts as a perfect agent, in the sense of choosing the quantities his patients demand at the user price. This ambiguity in the notion of agency means that welfare evaluations will often be ambiguous as well.

The Tasks of the Agent

I first indicate the problem that the consumer would like the physician acting as agent to solve. The consumer is initially assumed to maximize a utility function in health H and other goods X.

$$(1) \qquad U = U(X, H)$$

Other goods may be purchased at a price of one dollar, but health is not purchased directly. Rather, its production is given by:

$$(2) \qquad H = H_o + g(M; H_o)$$

where H_o is initial endowment of health, and M is a vector $M = (M_1, M_2, \ldots, M_n)$ of medical services. Time cost is ignored in this exposition; it can easily be added without altering conclusions. The vector of prices for medical care is P, and the consumer's income is Y. The consumer's problem is to maximize the utility function (1) subject to the production function constraint (2) and the income constraint

$$(3) \qquad Y = X + PM$$

Optimality requires that levels of medical inputs be chosen so that the marginal health products of a dollar spent on each are equal.

$$(4) \qquad \frac{\partial H / \partial M_1}{P_1} = \frac{\partial H / \partial M_2}{P_2} = \ldots = \frac{\partial H / \partial M_n}{P_n} = 1/\Pi$$

where Π is the shadow price (equal to marginal cost) of an increment in health. Optimality requires that the marginal rate of substitution between health and other goods equal its shadow price:

$$(5) \qquad \frac{U_H}{U_X} = \Pi$$

The vector M^* which satisfies (4) and (5) is the quantity the physician would choose if he were able and willing to act as a perfect agent. Note that this choice involves two subproblems. First, for whatever level of health produced, costs should be minimized (equation [4]). Second, the level of health should be that quantity that is demanded at the schedule of shadow prices (equation [5]). One may observe that the physician qua physician is more likely to have the knowledge needed to achieve (4) rather than (5), although even achievement of (4) requires that the physician know input prices as well as marginal effects on health.

Using the Model

From the utility function (1) and the constraints, it is obviously possible to derive a patient demand schedule for health as a function of the shadow price of health the patient faces. The shadow price in turn depends upon the price of health inputs and the patient's estimate of the marginal health products of those inputs. Given a homothetic production function, the mix of inputs chosen depends only on their relative marginal products and prices, not on the total amount of health demanded. The absolute level of marginal products determines the level of health the patient expects to achieve. Obviously, the information provided by the physician, or the choices that he makes, can reflect distorted relative *or* absolute health products.

Even if the physician is an income maximizer, he will act as the patient's agent in the sense of behaving in response to true relative marginal health products: he will minimize cost and will satisfy equation (4). But I also show that in his advice to the patient he would be expected to distort the absolute increase in health to be expected from a combination of medical inputs, and so he will not satisfy equation (5).

For simplicity, I begin by assuming that the physician maximizes his net money income. The health production function is altered to include explicitly two medical inputs. Input M_1 is produced by the physician (e.g., physician office visits) using his own time; M_1 is available at a constant marginal cost P_1. Input M_2 is sold at price P_2. No physician time is used in its production (e.g., prescription drugs or in-patient hospital care). In terms of the intermediate inputs M_1 and M_2, the health production function is:

$$H = H(M_1, M_2; H_o)$$

Suppose some increment to health $\Delta \bar{H}$ is to be produced. If the physician acts as a perfect agent, he will choose quantities ΔM_1 and ΔM_2 such that the ratios of their marginal products equal the ratios of their marginal costs. We may call these quantities M_1^* and M_2^*. Since the production function is assumed to be homothetic, $M_1^*/M_2^* = \bar{k}$, a constant given any level of relative prices.

The question now is whether the physician will choose the combination of inputs $\bar{k}$ if he acts to maximize his own income. We suppose that the patient as patient has no preferences as to the mix of medical care inputs, and regards the production function as a "black box"; he only cares about the health he will achieve and what he will have to spend to get it. The price he will have to pay for any batch of medical inputs is just the sum of their prices, but the health he expects to get depends in part on what the doctor tells him. However this expectation is formed, it does not, we assume, depend upon the mix or types of intermediate inputs. The patient views the physician as a prime contractor, who quotes him a total price and an expected final output. For a given expenditure, let the increment in health the physician tells the patient he will receive be $\Delta\hat{H}$; then the shadow price of a unit of health is approximately $\hat{\Pi} = \dfrac{P_1\Delta M_1 + P_2\Delta M_2}{\Delta\hat{H}}$. Obviously, the higher $\Delta\hat{H}$ the lower $\hat{\Pi}$ will be. The lower $\hat{\Pi}$, the more likely it is that the consumer will be willing to buy a larger number of units of health.

Consider first the situation in which the particular physician from whom the consumer purchases medical care is given, and the only question is how much the consumer will buy. If the physician is an income maximizer, he will set his price with regard to the patient's *total* demand curve for health. If he could get by with providing no inputs, he would set his price and choose what he would tell the patient so as to yield that shadow price for health which maximizes total revenue. If he must provide some inputs, for reasons to be suggested later, he would still maximize his income for any level of cost by representing $\Delta\hat{H}$ as greater than ΔH, i.e., by overstating the marginal health product of M. If, on the other hand, there is some competition among physicians and if the physician is a profit maximizer, his price will be set with regard to the *firm-level* demand curve for health. The physician will want to represent his performance of a particular procedure as likely to add as much or more health as performance of that procedure by any other physician.

Once the physician and patient agree on a total expenditure and an expected final level of health, we suppose that there must actually be some costs incurred and that there is some increment in health that must actually be delivered. In general, this actual level will differ from $\Delta\hat{H}$, but we suppose that it is determinate. It might be, for example, the minimum amount needed to forestall a malpractice suit, or undesirable competitive repercussions, or the consumer's prior knowledge might determine a maximum ratio of $\Delta\hat{H}$ to ΔH. With total expenditures already determined, and with the actual level of ΔH to be produced fixed by these minimal consumer expectations, physician income maximization will clearly require that the actual level of ΔH be produced in least-cost fashion. This is so even if some of the total expenditure goes for inputs which the physician himself does not employ, since the initial bargaining and information exchange only fixed the total expenditure for treatment, not its division among types of treatment. Were the physician to select anything other than the cost-minimizing input combination for whatever level of H he finally produces, he would reduce the amount he himself could collect. In summary, deviations from perfect agency would be limited to misrepresenting the marginal health product of care in general, and hence the shadow price of health.

Choice of Input Combinations in Practice

While it is a simple point that the income-maximizing physician will be likely to choose the cost-minimizing combination of inputs, it seems not to be recognized in much of the discussion of physician behavior, and in comparisons between that behavior under fee-for-service and prepaid group practice. Consider two kinds of other inputs: hospital admissions and prescription drugs. Both of these are almost always purchased (at least initially) in conjunction with physicians' services. Given a demand constraint (whether demand is competitive or not), the discussion above indicates that the maximizing physician has an incentive to choose the least-cost combination and type of inputs.

Yet it has often been alleged that such incentives are absent. For example, it has often been argued that physicians will tend to overuse hospital inputs primarily because they are "free." It is true that the cost of these inputs is not billed to the physician, but they are far from free if insurance coverage is not full. Of course, full insurance coverage makes them appear to be free, but this incentive would also appear in a prepaid group if it purchased its hospital insurance as a member of a large pool.

As another example, Victor Fuchs has stated, in connection with prescription drugs, "If (contrary to fact) the physician had a financial stake in keeping down the cost of drugs he prescribes, as he would under a comprehensive prepayment plan, he might be motivated to examine more closely drug prices and alternative products and he undoubtedly would also be less susceptible to persuasive detail men and high pressure advertising."[8] In fact, the physician *does* have a financial stake under an ideal fee-for-service market. Given the above formulation of demand, higher patient payments for prescription drugs reduce what the physician can charge for his own services. If the patient were willing to pay a higher price for, say, the more expensive branded drug the physician prescribed, he would also have been willing to pay the physician a higher fee. Indeed, the incentive to cost minimize is likely to be stronger at the level of the individual physician under fee-for-service than in a prepaid group, since a dollar in extra drug or hospital user costs reduces the fee-for-service physician's income by a full dollar, while in a typical prepaid practice the reduction in an individual physician's share would ordinarily be somewhat less.

All of this does not, of course, imply that actual choices one observes will be efficient; it only says that money income is maximized if they are efficient. If we look at studies of physicians' office practices, and examine how physicians use inputs for which they *do* pay directly, one generally finds that physicians have not made efficient choices. While there has not been much evidence of technical inefficiency, there is evidence that physicians do not use the net income-maximizing (or cost minimizing) number of aides.[9]

If physicians do not cost minimize in the choice of inputs in their own offices, one should probably not expect them to cost minimize in their choice of inputs elsewhere. Thus it seems to be very misleading to view such alleged inefficiencies as arising from the lack of financial incentives, or to view the prepaid group's incentive structure as something which would lead to improvement.

The question then becomes: Why do they not cost minimize? There are three possible explanations offered for the results in office practices. The first is that physicians do not know what the cost-minimizing combination is; for example, they mistakenly underestimate aide productivity. Usually it is not alleged that physicians are unaware of studies which show high aide productivity. Rather, they are held to be ignorant of how to use aide time efficiently in their own practices; they may not know how to delegate.

But this only appears to push the argument back a step. It is not that physicians underpurchase aides; it is that they underuse information on how to use aides. Welfare evaluation of such arguments is difficult, because of the problem of specifying the value of information when the buyer is intrinsically uncertain about what the information may tell him. Nevertheless, there appear to be no barriers to the spread of information on the use of aides. Such information is not generally of a public goods nature, since the physician would need to know how to use aides in his own practice. The probable reason why a physician has not experimented with more aides, and so does not know how to use them, is that the cost of experimentation exceeds the expected gains from future use of the aides. Similarly, the reason why physicians do not know when generic drugs are therapeutically equivalent to branded drugs is because the cost of the information is too great. Here the "information" is not generally the facts themselves, for those are reported in the *Medical Letter*, available at a nominal price. It is the cost of perusing and digesting this information. In summary, while lack of information may be a reason for nonuse of the least cost technique, it is not obvious that, when the costs of obtaining and processing information are added, the total costs of adopting and using the "least-cost" technique really are the lowest.

The second explanation is that output is measured improperly: a task performed by an aide really is not as productive or valuable as a task performed by a physician. While questionnaire surveys indicate that those patients who use services do not always feel this way, this question has never been answered definitively. It is hard to believe that, for tasks which involve diagnosis or judgment (as opposed to mechanical skill), a patient would not prefer a physician. Recent work by Coate on optometry, in which outputs can be measured much more easily, indicates little or no aide underuse.[10]

The third reason is that there are psychological costs to the monitoring and supervision of aides. Although monitoring an aide's performance may not take the physician more time, monitoring may take more effort or require him to reduce patient contact in which he takes pleasure. He may simply not prefer to work in the style of practice associated with larger numbers of aides; there is little in the process of physician selection, training, or continuing education which is likely to result in high levels of skill in personnel management. This last reason may be a plausible explanation for the observed facts: physicians do not choose the cheapest drug *or* the ideal number of aides because they do not want to take the effort to seek the most efficient method of practice.

It is important to recognize the welfare implications of this explanation: if these costs do exist, it is *not* necessarily inefficient to do the inefficient thing. Put differently, the compensation that physicians would have to be paid to induce them to search out the cheapest drug or make the effort to supervise aides would exceed the cost savings to be realized. Put still differently, a rule which required physicians to use the optimal number of aides, or search for the cheapest drug, might indeed reduce costs. But it would make physicians worse off. The amount physicians might be willing to pay to remove the rule might exceed the amount of cost saving. Distributional questions aside, "efficiency" is not necessarily desirable; psychic costs are not imaginary; they are as real as the value of leisure time that the worker gives up or the enjoyment of goods and services that a consumer must sacrifice. The utility-maximizing behavior of physicians may make this case differ from the normal one of joint products. Utility maximization by physicians, as suppliers and managers, may indeed make medical services in general, and prescription drugs in particular, different from furniture or automobiles.

There is, of course, a distributional effect, a question of property rights. Forcing physicians to do the efficient thing may permit the class of consumers to be better off, but it makes physicians worse off. More to the point, the amount by which physicians are made worse off exceeds the amount by which consumers are made better off. The class of physicians could offer a bribe to consumers *not* to impose "efficiency" rules on them which would exceed the gains consumers might expect from increased efficiency. The fairytale character of this political fable suggests that we might expect such "efficiency" rules to be imposed even if they are inefficient, just because consumers are more numerous (though perhaps not always more politically potent) than physicians.

Unequal Information, or A Little Knowledge Can Be a Dangerous Thing

In the preceding discussion I assumed that the individual consumer determined how much medical care to buy in total, and how much to buy from each provider, on the basis of the total price (over all inputs) that he would have to pay for an increment of health. The consumer was assumed to pay no attention either to the mix or to the prices of individual intermediate inputs. There are two possible objections to this assumption. First, individuals may judge the health outcomes they expect to receive not just by what the physician tells them, but by the actual intermediate inputs provided. If consumers think they will be more likely to recover with a branded drug than a generic one, or with any prescription at all (even an unnecessary one), rather than just advice and hand-holding, then obviously the cost-minimizing mix of inputs may not maximize physician income. Income-maximizing physicians may find it worthwhile to cater to uninformed consumer desires. Second, and possibly more important, it is plausible to conjecture that the elasticity of demand for health from a given provider may not be the same for all input mixes. (Even if this elasticity were the same, of course, the elasticities of demand for individual inputs would generally differ. Doubling the surgeon's fee will generally have less effect on the demand for hospital admissions than would doubling the hospital price, even given equal insurance coverage.) Differences may arise because the consumer has different amounts of information about the prices and practices of various physicians.

Concretely, consumers may have a rough idea of what a physician's fee for an office visit ought to be. Suppose the consumer has some information about the going prices for routine physician services. He knows that an office visit typically costs between $10 and $20. He has very little information on the prices, types, and quantities of prescription drugs provided for various illnesses, or the usefulness of hospitalization or laboratory tests in connection with a particular illness. Suppose that physicians in his area typically order $30 worth of diagnostic tests for a particular condition, and charge $15 for an office visit. Suppose the tests are in fact worthless, or nearly so. By the argument in the section "Using the Model," each physician would have an incentive to stop ordering the test, thus saving the patient $30, and raising his fee to capture some of the gains from not prescribing the test. Suppose a particular physician raised his office fee to \$30, and prescribed no tests. Under full information this would attract patients to him, since his cost for treating the illness is \$30, as opposed to \$45 total cost for other physicians. But if consumers do not observe the total cost, but only the \$30 versus \$15 difference in office fees, this cost-minimizing physician may actually lose patients even while making them better off.

More formally, the problem is that, if information differs in this way, the firm-level demand elasticity may be smaller with respect to the prices of the "ordered" inputs than with respect to the physician's own input. While the physician would have an incentive to inform patients of his low-cost mode of treatment (and many do), this ability is limited by restrictions on advertising and the heterogeneity of treatment modes. An interesting empirical question would be whether the elasticities do differ in this way.

A second possibility is that, however desirable it might be, the physician may be unable to vary his own charge. This may happen because of third party reimbursement arrangements or because of price controls. However desirable price limitation may be for other reasons, it does have the effect of eliminating any cost-minimization incentive to the physician who does not have excess capacity, for he will be unable to capture any cost savings in his own fee. If he is willing to supply more output at the going price than is demanded of him, then he may be able to increase the quantity demanded from him by lowering the cost of other inputs.

Conclusion

That physicians only direct rather than pay for many other health inputs need not lead to departures from cost-minimizing behavior. This conclusion holds even though physicians may be able to induce consumers to obtain amounts of health, and consequently amounts of medical care services of all types, that differ from those that would have been provided were consumers not ignorant. How consumers decide how much to believe of what physicians tell them and how their beliefs affect their consumption decisions and constrain the actions of physicians will be treated in more detail in subsequent chapters.

2 Physicians and Hospitals

Many physicians do not produce the bulk of their output in their own offices, where they pay the outlay costs of inputs used. Instead, much of their output is produced in the hospital, where they neither have ownership rights nor are directly responsible for paying the cost of hospital inputs.

The preceding chapter suggested that, if physicians were income maximizers, we should expect them to use an efficient combination of inputs, whether or not they made explicit outlays for those inputs. If they were utility maximizers, no alternative institutional arrangement could improve efficiency. Yet it is widely suggested that hospitals are inefficient, even though the empirical (as opposed to anecdotal) evidence for this contention is weak, and there is some evidence that very little of the interhospital variation in hospital costs can be attributed to inefficiency.[1] It is also not generally recognized that efficiency cannot be judged solely by the costs the hospital pays, but must also include consideration of the cost of inputs supplied by physicians. Consequently, it remains to investigate whether there are any reasons to suppose that physicians will not, individually and collectively, use hospital inputs efficiently.

There are two broad classes of reasons we will consider. Both reasons are based on distortions in the prices physicians-as-agents face for hospital inputs. Those distortions may arise either from (1) customary forms of hospitalization insurance or (2) from imperfect cooperation of physicians within the hospital, aggravated by imperfect pricing of hospital services. Each of these reasons will be considered in turn.

Hospitalization Insurance

Typical hospitalization insurance in the United States makes payments to hospitals which depend on the hospital costs or bills incurred by

17

insureds. It is easy to see intuitively that this arrangement will induce physicians to choose higher levels of costly hospital inputs than would occur without insurance, as long as that cost is associated with improvement in patient well-being. Because the user cost of an increment in quality will have been reduced by insurance, patients, or their physicians acting as agents, will tend to choose higher quality. Because there may be a time cost associated with increased quantity (in the sense of patient-days), but no time cost for additional quality or services during a day the patient is already in the hospital, one would expect the response of quality to insurance to be greater than the response of quantity. Of course, increased quality will show up as higher costs or charges per unit output. In demanding higher quality for his patients, each physician is acting as their true agent, even though the result for all patients of all physicians is likely to be inefficient. This type of "moral hazard" has generally been recognized as an important determinant of hospital cost inflation, and does not require further discussion here.[2] Virtually complete insurance coverage also reduces the incentive for patient or physician to search for lower cost or more efficient hospitals, and can thereby contribute to inflation.[3]

There is another less obvious but possibly important effect of typical hospitalization insurance. Such insurance will tend to encourage excessive substitution of hospital inputs for physician inputs. This oversubstitution not only causes the hospital unit cost to rise, but total costs per unit (over hospitals and physicians) rise as well: there will be overuse of hospital inputs relative to physician inputs, as compared to the cost-minimizing level.

To see this, suppose that, in the absence of insurance, the equilibrium gross price of hospital output at a given hospital is $\bar{P}_T$, and the quality $\bar{Q}$. $\bar{P}_T$ is the sum of the hospital price $\bar{P}_H$ and the physician price $\bar{P}_M$. Assume for simplicity that the price $\bar{P}_T$ is competitively determined; permitting the extent of competition to vary with the level of insurance coverage would unnecessarily complicate the problem. Suppose there is an opportunity cost C of physician time spent in the hospital; this could be either the physician's income from providing ambulatory care or a money measure of his value of leisure. Suppose the only hospital input is represented by H, which is available at a constant unit cost W. Finally, suppose that the hospital price P_H is set equal to average cost: $P_H = WH/Q$. Holding output constant at, say, $\bar{Q}$, it is possible to substitute H for M within the limits given by

$$\frac{\partial Q}{\partial H} dH - \frac{\partial Q}{\partial M} dM = 0$$

Cost minimization for a given output implies that

$$\frac{W}{\partial Q/\partial H} = \frac{C}{\partial Q/\partial M}$$

Let H^* and M^* be the levels of M and H which satisfy this equality. It follows that if H is increased by a small amount ΔH, and M is reduced to $M^* - \Delta M$, Q constant, then

$$W\Delta H \simeq C\Delta M$$

The reduction in physician opportunity cost would approximately equal the increase in hospital cost.

Now suppose that there exists an insurance which covers $\lambda(0 > \lambda > 1)$ of P_H. The insured pays $(1-\lambda)(P_H) + P_M$ for a unit of hospital care instead of $\bar{P}_H + \bar{P}_M$. If, after the provision of insurance, output is to be held constant at $\bar{Q}$, the physician price must rise by λP_H to keep price constant at $\bar{P}_T$. Physician income will then increase by $\bar{Q}(\lambda P_H)$.

Suppose H is increased by ΔH and M decreased by ΔM as before. The rise in the use of hospital inputs raises P_H by $W\Delta H/Q$. In order to keep the user price constant at $\bar{P}_T$, the physician price will have to fall by $(1-\lambda)W\Delta H/Q$, and physician gross revenues by $(1-\lambda)W\Delta H$. The reduction in physician opportunity cost is $C\Delta M$. Since initially $C\Delta M \simeq W\Delta H$, it follows that $C\Delta M > (1-\lambda)W\Delta H$. That is, the decline in physician costs $(-C\Delta M)$ exceeds the decline in physician gross revenues $\{(1-\lambda)W\Delta H\}$. So physician net income will increase if the level of physician input is reduced while the level of hospital inputs is increased. Of course, equilibrium output will also change, and may be accompanied by changes in input ratios, but it will still be true that, whatever level of output is produced, it will be produced with relatively more than the cost-minimizing amount of H. With hospitalization insurance, substitution of hospital for physician inputs increases total cost, but it also increases total revenue by several times the increase in total cost, enough to offset the increase in total cost. Put still another way, hospital insurance reduces the user price of hospital inputs below their "true" market price, and so leads to the use of relatively more of them.

Physician Fee Insurance

Where hospitalization insurance is present, insurance to cover physician charges for in-hospital physician services is also typically found. This result should not be surprising: if the loss from consuming one more unit of hospital output is the total price $P_M + P_H$, then one would expect to find both parts of the hospital bill covered by insurance. Would insurance coverage of the physician's fee offset the incentive to

overuse of hospital inputs? To answer this question, we need to consider two kinds of physician fee insurance.

1. "Indemnity" insurance. Many physician insurance policies pay the
entire physician's bill or a maximum dollar amount, whichever is less.
Sometimes the maximum is set by an explicit schedule of maximum fees,
although more recently it has been set at some percentile of a screen of
reasonable and customary fees. We shall consider first the situations in
which the full maximum amount is paid.

Under such an arrangement, the insurance payment is independent
of both the level of the physician's fee (once it is at or above the maximum) and the way the physician uses his time. It is obvious that such
insurance coverage will not affect the relative use of inputs, since the
insurance payment does not depend on the amount of inputs used.

2. Proportional coinsurance. When the fee is below the fee schedule
maximum, then insurance coverage may have some effect if the insur-
ance pays some fraction $\gamma \leq 1$ of the fee. If γ is less than one, holding
P_T constant implies that P_M is increased to $\dfrac{1}{(1-\gamma)} P_M$ when insurance is
obtained. Ideally, P_T could still be held constant by raising P_M by this
amount, reducing P_H, and continuing to use the cost-minimizing combination of inputs. However, the hospital would then sustain a deficit,
and there might be practical problems getting physicians to underwrite
this deficit.

If the hospital is constrained to charge a breakeven price, physician
insurance may provide an incentive to reduce hospital inputs. Reducing
hospital inputs and raising the physician's fee (and his time inputs) may
lead to higher physician net incomes as long as the rise in the physician
fee exceeds the opportunity cost of the extra physician time.

The conclusion is that *some* physician insurance schemes may produce an offsetting effect. But since in any market area many persons
with hospital insurance will not have physician insurance with the proportional coinsurance type of coverage, the effect of hospital insurance
on input combinations will not be fully offset.[4]

Imperfect Pricing, Imperfect Cooperation, and the Size Principle

If all hospital services were sold at the marginal cost of the inputs
used to produce those services, and if insurance were not present, physicians would have an incentive to minimize total costs. The physician
would know that any extra hospital inputs he ordered would show up
on a hospital bill to his patient, which would mean less that he could
collect. The cost-minimizing solution would be chosen by the physician
because prices would play the role of coordinator. In such a situation,
the physician would not treat the hospital as a rent-free workshop,
despite the nominal separation of physician and hospital billing.

But there are reasons to expect that hospitals cannot or will not price every dimension of their service at its marginal cost, and so will offer another incentive to the physician to depart from the cost-minimizing input combination. First, pricing at marginal cost may involve enormous administrative problems in monitoring every extra nursing or house-keeping minute devoted to each patient. And second, even if pricing at marginal cost were feasible, it might cause the hospital to violate the zero profit constraint when marginal and average costs diverge. In particular, if there are services which involve high initial fixed costs, pricing at marginal cost may not permit the hospital to cover costs and still provide all services which generate consumers' surplus.

Even with average cost pricing, there will still be some incentive for the physician to keep costs down, since the individual physician will bear some fraction of any addition to total costs he might cause. But the larger the number of physicians over whose patients these costs are spread, the smaller will be the share and the smaller the incentive for each individual physician. This "size principle" has been extensively discussed in the literature.[5]

One would expect physicians collectively to try to institute some means of enforcing cooperation. This might take the form of rules, committee structures, moral suasion, and so on. They may delegate some of this task to the hospital's lay administration or to chiefs of the medical service. One would also expect physicians to sort themselves according to their responsiveness to incentives, or their degree of cooperativeness. But eventually there will be some departure from the perfectly cooperative, cost-minimizing solution, if only because coordination is itself costly.

This departure from cost-minimization will take two forms. Both of them will involve reduction in the amount of physician inputs, but they differ with regard to the type of input whose amount is altered. The physician provides two inputs to the medical care process: his own time and what one might call "effort" or care in directing the production process. Imperfect cooperation can affect the amounts of both of these inputs.

When the physician or his patient bears only a partial share of the benefit from his being careful and being concerned about the costliness of treatment procedures, and when such effort or care involves disutility, one would expect to observe less effort and higher hospital costs than when the physician can receive the full reward from "effort." The physician's physical time input will also be lower, and hospital costs higher, when the physician cannot capture all of the benefit from devoting his own time to hospital care. If he values his time in other activities, one would expect him to order hospital substitutes for it to a greater extent as the fraction he receives of the benefit from the increased productivity of that time input becomes smaller. The result would be an overuse of hospital input relative to physician input. Because hospitals price many services on an average cost basis, as noted above, one would therefore expect some overuse of hospital inputs (relative to physician inputs) to occur.

Because effort or care cannot be measured directly, the first effect is much more difficult to determine.[6] However, the second type of overuse is one that can be detected directly by measuring physician time input. It is this second type that will be investigated in the empirical work in the following chapter.

This discussion is based on a model of the hospital in which physicians control the hospital, and induce it to operate so as to maximize their individual utilities, even though they may be constrained by problems of size and coordination. The alternative "hospital administration utility-maximization" models developed by Feldstein and Newhouse make no direct prediction about physician-hospital input ratios, since they do not treat nonsalaried physician time as a productive input.[7] The result of overuse of hospital relative to physician input would, however, be consistent with their kind of theory if higher "quality" were equated with more hospital and less physician input. Whether hospital administrators, who run the hospital according to the theory, actually judge quality in this way or not is unknown.

Measuring Input Substitution in Practice

The way in which inputs are to be measured when estimating a production function depends upon the use to which the results are to be put. In engineering, where it is the purely technical relationships that are of interest, the most appropriate measure would be some index of homogeneous productive effort. If, on the other hand, one is interested in the behavioral response of the system, the appropriate measure is the level of input that can be manipulated by the decision-maker. In more concrete terms, whether one wishes to measure labor input by minutes actually worked at various tasks or by hours of work for which full wages are received depends upon whether or not a feasible control mechanism exists for monitoring, controlling, and paying for only minutes of actual work. Even this states the matter too simply, since what is feasible may often be too costly, and the actual methods of control and reimbursement (and hence the actual allocation of effort) may vary widely among occupations, firms, or skill levels.

All this discussion is by way of elaborate rationalization for the use, in the production function estimates that follow, of the number of physicians available to provide care, rather than actual hours worked, as a measure of physician input. The concrete reason for this procedure is the unavailability of hours-worked data, but the reason for continuing with the analysis is that, at the present time, the most that might be manipulable from a public policy viewpoint is the number of physicians in an area or on a hospital staff, *not* the number of hours the physician spends at the hospital. In general, the kind of question to be posed is: If one pours additional physicians into a hospital's catchment area, or places additional physicians on its staff, what effect will this have, *ceteris paribus*, on the hospital's output? Put another way, the question is that of how physicians affect hospital productivity.

While allegations of physician overuse of hospital inputs are common, concrete descriptions of the form this overuse might take are less common. The possibility of overuse is most transparent for hospital-employed physicians: they can be substituted for the time of private practice physicians, and one suspects that there is not an off-setting diminution in fees charged by the private practice physician. A similar argument might be made with respect to nurses; they can perform actions which can save the attending physician the time and trouble of making a visit to the patient. The argument that when nurses are scarce, physicians will end up making more visits is a little weaker, but perhaps plausible, especially if one adds the notion of "highly skilled" nurses.

Another way in which physicians substitute for hospital inputs has been suggested by Martin Feldstein: "By increasing the number of doctors, for instance, a hospital may be able to shorten the length of patient stay and thus decrease the input of beds for a given output."[8] While Feldstein's study referred to hospitals in the United Kingdom, the same sort of reasoning might be applied to hospitals in the United States, and to other hospital inputs (nurses, for instance) as well. The explanation here would seem to be that either rate of recovery or delay in performing procedures can be affected by the number of physicians. Where the number of medical staff members are few, rounds may be less frequent, and patients may have to wait in bed for the physician to come by and order procedures, perform operations, or sign discharge forms. I shall later try to determine whether any effect of physicians on output does come through on effect on length of stay.

It should be emphasized that, inasmuch as the estimates to be presented are production function estimates, they do not bear directly on the question of whether physicians can create demand for hospital services. As in other production function studies, we do not ask whether the output should have been produced, or why it was produced; we only ask about the relationship between outputs and inputs. These results do, however, bear indirectly on the question of demand creation, in that they indicate the maximum extent of demand creation, at least as far as physicians are directly concerned. In other words, they indicate the maximum amount of increase in output that could be attributed to demand creation by additional physicians when all hospital inputs are held constant. However, since inputs and outputs are not measured in per capita terms, the results are not directly comparable to those from demand studies.

One difficulty with the empirical analysis is that scale or hospital size is likely to be positively correlated with the number of physicians and with the level of physician input. Hospitals with larger medical staffs will have more physician time input available, but more difficulty in coordinating it. In such a case it is not possible to get separate estimates of "true" economies of scale *and* the effects of the size principle. If it were possible to measure physician time directly, and observe situations in which different numbers of physicians provide the same amount of time, then one could get a separate estimate of the effect of the size principle.

Conclusion

The following chapter presents production function estimates intended to measure the existence and extent of underuse of physician input. Unfortunately, available data do not permit an explanation of the cause of departures from optimal use; we do not have measures of the extent of insurance coverage or of departures from marginal cost pricing.

3 Physician Influence on the Productivity of Hospitals: Empirical Results

Do physicians in fact choose the level of their own inputs and the inputs provided by the hospital in the way described in the preceding chapter? Do they cause the overuse of hospital inputs relative to physician inputs? This chapter presents the results of an empirical estimation of a hospital production function for a set of hospitals in the United States. The data contain a measure of physician inputs, and make possible some answers to these questions.

The Sample

A sample of 165 predominantly rural counties in 9 midwestern states was selected. Each of these counties had just one short-term general hospital with more than 50 beds throughout the period 1966–72. It is reasonable to suppose that the great bulk of hospital care provided by physicians in each county was provided at the sample hospital. The intent was to choose approximately 50 hospitals in each of four categories: not-for-profit, 50–100 beds in 1966; governmental 50–100 beds in 1966; not-for-profit, over 100 beds; and governmental, over 100 beds. There was not a sufficiently large number of hospitals with reasonably complete data in the third and fourth categories to permit 50 observations, the second category was slightly oversampled, and later editing reduced the sample size in all categories. However, since the sample was nonrandom to begin with, these characteristics did not seem to justify a complex procedure of stratifying or replacing observations excluded by editing, which would have required adding observations from non-midwestern states. The editing consisted of removing hospitals for which data were missing, and removing one hospital which, although classified in 1966 as short-term, changed to long-term in subsequent years. Data on these hospitals for 1966–72 were obtained from the American Hospital Association *Annual Survey of Hospitals.* In order to obtain a proxy measure for the amount of physician input in hospitals for each of these counties, the American Medical Association's Distribution of Physicians data were used to list the number of patient care physicians of various types in each county. The measure of physician input used was therefore a measure of the number of physicians available for patient care in the county. This was obviously not the measure of physician input most desirable for production function estimates. However, it is *the level of input that is likely to be manipulable by policy.* That is, public policy has been and is generally directed at getting more physicians to locate in rural areas. It is not directed at controlling the allocation of their time. The results show what may be expected in terms of hospital output by adding or removing physicians who treat their patients at that hospital.

Hospital staff appointments are not at present a matter of public policy, but the development of policy on such matters is not inconceivable. For a single year (1972), I obtained data from the Social Security Administration's "Provider of Services" file on the number of staff physicians at each of the sample hospitals, and on a finer breakdown of nonphysician personnel into categories. These data are provided periodically by all participating hospitals as part of the Medicare certification program.

Functional Forms

A Cobb-Douglas function is probably the most convenient functional form to use in estimating production functions. Whether it is appropriate is another matter. One problem that arose in Reinhardt's study of physician input into the production of ambulatory care[1] is not present here. In the physician's office, output can be produced even if no aides are employed, but the Cobb-Douglas function requires that all inputs be positive if output is to be positive. The four inputs that are used in most of the estimates are hospital beds, nonphysician hospital personnel (full-time equivalents), other nonlabor hospital inputs (meals, drugs, etc.) and physicians. Each of these would appear to be essential, and each is positive in all of the sample hospitals. Hence, the requirement of the Cobb-Douglas form that every input be positive is not onerous. A more serious restriction of the Cobb-Douglas form is that it constrains the elasticity of substitution to unity. Other forms are available which do not require this constraint, but their use raises more complex estimation problems. Since we do not know a priori whether the Cobb-Douglas form is reasonable or not, I have followed Feldstein in first estimating that form, and then considering alternative specifications only if the

Cobb-Douglas form appears "unreasonable." Judgment is obviously involved here.[2]

When physicians or personnel are disaggregated into specialty types, zero values for inputs do occur. Results are obtained both using the Cobb-Douglas functional form but with a positive constant (one) added to all values of these variables, and using the "transcendental" form suggested by Reinhardt.[3]

Variables

For the cross section 1966–72, and for the pooled cross sections, values of both beds and personnel were taken from the American Hospital Association's *Guide Issue*. A variable to represent nonlabor inputs other than beds was constructed by subtracting from nonlabor expense the product ($BEDS \times 1000$), where $1000 is an estimate of the annual depreciation expense per bed on beds alone. Sensitivity of the results to this assumption will be discussed below. Output was defined as the number of cases treated, as measured by the number of admissions. While it would have been desirable to have an explicit measure of casemix, such data were not available. Because the sample hospitals are the sole hospitals serving relatively similar populations and are not major teaching hospitals, variation in casemix is not likely to be great. The output of the hospital is assumed to be a "treated case." Each case, it is assumed, is treated to the same degree; quality is assumed to be unrelated to input mix, and days of stay are assumed *not* to be of value in themselves. Fuchs has noted that it is not even clear whether additional days of stay should be treated as beneficial, because they mean more bed and board, or as detrimental, because they delay the patient's resumption of normal activities.[4] The actual estimating equations were of the form

$$lnADMISSIONS = a_o + \beta_1 \, lnBEDS + \beta_2 \, lnPERSNL + \beta_3 \, lnMD + \beta_4 \, lnNLIP + \gamma \, TIME + u$$

where   *ADMISSIONS* is inpatient admissions per year;

                BEDS is short term beds available;

                PERSNL is full-time-equivalent nonphysician personnel;

                MD is medical staff measures;

                NLIP is a nonlabor inputs measure; and

                TIME is time, measured from 1 to 7.

Results

Table 3.1 indicates the results using total patient care physicians (*MD*) as a measure of physician input, and hospital full-time-equivalent nonphysician personnel as a measure of the nonphysician labor input. The coefficient on the physician input, the elasticity of admissions with respect to the number of physicians in the county, is always significant, at the 0.01 level or better, and in the range of 0.11 to 0.17.[5] Personnel and nonlabor expense are likewise always significant. Measured hospital productivity decreased during this period at a rate of about 3% per year. It is likely that this decline in measured productivity captures increases in the service intensity or style of care, especially since actual admissions were increasing on average at these hospitals. The *BEDS* variable is significant only for nonprofit hospitals; except for this difference, the production function does not appear to differ across hospital types. Not-for-profit hospitals above 100 beds and large hospitals overall display approximately constant returns to scale, while for all other hospital

Table 3.1   Production Function Estimates: All M.D.'s Dependent Variable: Admissions

Sample	Con-stant	Beds	Person-nel	M.D.'s	Non-labor input	Time	Σ Co-effs.	n	$\bar{R}^2$
Full	3.9	.086	.52	.15	.15	−.029	.904	1145	.864
Sample		(2.7)	(16.4)	(10.7)	(8.7)	(7.7)	(41.1)		
Beds>100	3.7	.16	.49	.16	.14	−.030	.941	421	.857
		(3.3)	(10.2)	(3.3)	(4.9)	(5.1)	(29.2)		
Beds:	4.2	.002	.53	.13	.15	−.027	.810	724	.658
50–100		(0.1)	(12.1)	(6.0)	(7.3)	(5.3)	(32.7)		
Govern-	3.9	.00	.57	.14	.17	−.031	.873	615	.807
mental		(0.01)	(11.0)	(6.2)	(5.2)	(6.2)	(19.7)		
Not-for-	3.8	.18	.45	.17	.13	−.030	.934	530	.907
profit		(4.0)	(11.2)	(10.0)	(6.7)	(6.1)	(40.0)		
NFP,	3.6	.28	.37	.16	.16	−.032	.979	240	.877
Beds>100		(4.5)	(6.0)	(6.8)	(4.2)	(4.3)	(33.8)		
NFP, Beds	4.1	.091	.50	.17	.12	−.027	.878	291	.700
50–100		(1.6)	(9.5)	(5.8)	(5.3)	(4.0)	(32.0)		
Govt.	3.9	.004	.62	.15	.11	−.026	.888	181	.800
Beds>100		(0.0)	(8.5)	(3.7)	(2.2)	(2.9)	(16.3)		
Govt. Beds	4.3	−.057	.53	.11	.19	−.032	.778	434	.637
50–100		(0.9)	(8.0)	(3.9)	(5.2)	(4.3)	(13.1)		
Occup.	3.9	.065	.47	.17	.19	−.032	.898	463	.887
>75%		(1.4)	(9.2)	(7.4)	(6.1)	(4.8)	(49.9)		
Full	3.5	.088	.64	—	.18	−.041	.904	1145	.849
Sample		(2.6)	(19.3)	—	(7.2)	(10.0)	(60.0)		

NOTE: *t* ratios in parentheses.

Table 3.2   **Sample Means and Standard Deviations**

Sample	Hos- pitals	Beds	Per- sonnel	M.D.'s	NLIP ($ thou.)	G.P.'s	Surg. spec.	Med. spec.	Other spec.	Hosp. based phys.
Full	165	108	190	17.4	491	9.3	3.7	1.8	1.8	0.7
Sample		(60)	(127)	(15.4)	(435)	(5.1)	(4.9)	(3.3)	(3.1)	(2.1)
Beds	60	158	292	28.3	777	11.8	7.3	4.0	3.7	1.5
>100		(70)	(154)	(20.4)	(561)	(6.5)	(6.4)	(4.5)	(4.3)	(3.2)
Beds	105	78	131	11.1	325	7.9	1.6	0.5	0.7	0.3
50–100		(24)	(46)	(4.9)	(202)	(3.3)	(1.5)	(0.9)	(1.1)	(0.7)
Govt.	88	97	171	15.3	432	9.3	2.9	1.2	1.4	0.6
		(45)	(45)	(10.7)	(335)	(4.6)	(3.2)	(2.2)	(2.3)	(1.2)
Not-for-	77	119	212	19.8	560	9.4	4.7	2.5	2.3	0.9
Profit		(72)	(153)	(19.2)	(519)	(5.6)	(6.2)	(4.1)	(3.8)	(2.8)
NFP Beds:	35	168	315	30.8	860	11.4	8.4	4.9	4.3	1.7
>100		(80)	(174)	(23.9)	(621)	(7.0)	(7.5)	(5.1)	(4.8)	(4.0)
NFP Beds:	42	79	127	10.8	312	7.8	1.6	0.5	0.7	0.3
50–100		(22)	(42)	(4.6)	(194)	(3.3)	(1.5)	(0.7)	(1.0)	(0.5)
Govt. Beds	26	143	262	25.1	666	12.4	5.9	2.8	3.0	1.1
>100		(48)	(117)	(13.7)	(449)	(5.8)	(4.2)	(3.2)	(3.2)	(1.4)
Govt. Beds	62	78	133	11.2	334	8.0	1.7	0.6	0.7	0.3
50–100		(26)	(48)	(5.1)	(206)	(3.2)	(1.5)	(1.0)	(1.2)	(0.9)
Occ. >	66	120	229	22.1	596	10.3	5.3	2.9	2.6	1.0
75%		(76)	(161)	(20.3)	(524)	(5.9)	(6.4)	(4.3)	(4.1)	(2.9)

NOTE: Standard deviations are in parentheses.

subsamples, and for the full sample, the sum of coefficients is significantly less than unity, indicating decreasing returns.

The most likely reason for the insignificance of beds is the high correlation of this variable with personnel ($r = .91$). High multicollinearity is to be expected in production function estimates; perhaps its existence might also explain why Feldstein's results for British hospitals were "unreasonable," with low or insignificant coefficients for such obviously important inputs as nurses. Heteroskedasticity was anticipated, but did not occur; error variances were almost identical for each quartile.

There is a potential problem in the estimates because of the possibility of excess capacity. The possibility of excess capacity in any of the inputs is disturbing in any production function study. It is even more disturbing here because the measured amount of the physician input may well be correlated with the extent of excess capacity in the other inputs. If it is supposed that hospitals may have excess capacity in the hospital inputs (beds, personnel, and other nonlabor inputs), and if physicians can in part create or activate demand for hospital care, then it is possible that any observed increase in output related to the presence of larger numbers of physicians, observed hospital inputs held constant,

Table 3.3   Population Rates: Sample Means and Standard Deviations

Sample	Popu-lation (00)	Adm. Pop.	M.D. Pop.	Person-nel Pop.	Beds Pop.	G.P.'s Pop.	Surg. Pop.
Full	283	14.4	0.060	0.75	0.45	0.036	0.012
	(185)	(6.5)	(0.025)	(0.35)	(0.23)	(0.013)	(0.012)
Beds	402	16.0	0.072	0.85	0.48	0.031	0.019
>100	(238)	(7.3)	(0.029)	(0.40)	(0.27)	(0.011)	(0.015)
Beds:	214	13.5	0.054	0.69	0.43	0.039	0.008
50–100	(94)	(5.8)	(0.019)	(0.31)	(0.21)	(0.013)	(0.009)
Govt.	271	13.7	0.057	0.70	0.41	0.036	0.010
	(164)	(6.5)	(0.022)	(0.33)	(0.19)	(0.011)	(0.011)
Not-for-	297	15.2	0.065	0.80	0.49	0.035	0.014
profit	(208)	(6.4)	(0.027)	(0.37)	(0.27)	(0.014)	(0.013)
NFP Beds:	403	17.2	0.076	0.93	0.53	0.030	0.021
>100	(251)	(7.6)	(0.032)	(0.42)	(0.31)	(0.012)	(0.015)
NFP Beds:	208	13.5	0.055	0.69	0.45	0.040	0.008
50–100	(99)	(4.6)	(0.016)	(0.27)	(0.21)	(0.014)	(0.008)
Govt. Beds:	399	14.3	0.066	0.74	0.42	0.033	0.016
>100	(220)	(6.6)	(0.024)	(0.33)	(0.18)	(0.010)	(0.013)
Govt. Beds:	218	13.4	0.053	0.68	0.41	0.038	0.008
50–100	(90)	(6.4)	(0.020)	(0.33)	(0.20)	(0.012)	(0.010)
Occ. >	336	14.8	0.064	0.76	0.42	0.034	0.014
75%	(233)	(7.3)	(0.029)	(0.37)	(0.20)	(0.011)	(0.015)

NOTE: Rates are rates per 100 persons.

may not in fact reflect physician input productivity. Instead, we may only be observing more intensive use of previously underutilized hospital inputs. As noted in the preceding chapter, this problem cannot be fully resolved without direct measurement of underused inputs. Even if physician inputs actually rise, the total change in hospital output would be the sum of the direct effect of physician inputs, holding the utilization or service flow of hospital inputs constant, *plus* the increase in output arising from the greater flows of productive services from the hospital inputs. There is, of course, some ambiguity in the notion of excess capacity, and some question of how to measure it and incorporate it into production function estimates.

In order to determine whether the estimates presented above might be affected by this excess capacity effect, it is useful to determine whether the measured effect of physicians on output varies with the level of hospital excess capacity. The lower the level of excess capacity, the closer the coefficient on physicians will approximate the true output elasticity. The average occupancy rate of all hospitals in the sample is about 70%. A subsample of these hospitals with occupancy rates (in any year) greater than 75% was selected.[6] The estimated production function is shown in the second to last line of table 3.1. The values of coefficients on all variables, including physicians, are practically unchanged from the full sample results. These results suggest that the presence of excess capacity does not bias the coefficient estimates. Of course, if additional physicians mean *no* physician input, or if none of the hospitals ever reaches a capacity constraint at any time during the year, then this argument does not hold. Neither of these suppositions seems plausible.

Finally, comparison of the first and last lines in table 3.1 indicates that omission of the physician input did not bias estimates of returns to scale. Omission of the physician input does, however, lead to an overestimate of both the effect of personnel on output and of the rate of decrease in productivity over time. Adding the physician input makes only a modest contribution to the explanatory power of the regression, as might be expected given the high multicollinearity of the input variables.

Table 3.4 shows the result of a similar estimate using disaggregated measures of physician input. (For each of these physician measures, a constant (1) was added to prevent zero observations). The explanatory power of the regression is not appreciably improved by this change, but the results do shed some light on the way hospital output responds to subspecialties.[7] (The coefficient on the time variable is almost the same as in table 3.1, and so is omitted.) Not surprisingly, hospital based specialists, uncommon in hospitals under 100 beds anyway, tend to depress output there, probably because their presence is a proxy for case complexity. Similarly, medical specialists (internists, pediatricians, etc.) tend to affect output only in the large hospitals. Both surgical specialists and G.P.'s have positive output elasticities everywhere. Interpretation of the coefficients on G.P.'s and surgeons can be simplified by converting the elasticities into marginal products per physician. Table 3.5 shows that the marginal product of a physician is about 35 admissions per year, or about 3 per month. As might be expected, the marginal product is higher for surgeons than G.P.'s, and the difference tends to widen in the larger hospitals and counties where specialization by surgeons may occur to a greater extent. The purely hospital based physicians have a high marginal product in the larger hospitals.

Since many of the measures of input used here are obviously very crude, it seems appropriate to test the sensitivity of the results to alternative measures. Table 3.6 presents the results of such tests.

Output has been measured by the admission or case treated. I have argued that "quality" or casemix is not likely to differ in a systematic way across the sample hospitals, since the hospitals are stratified by size and since the populations served are all from relatively rural midwestern counties. One attempt to control for "quality" would be by introducing the number of approvals (of education programs) and accreditations, as well as the number of facilities at the hospital as independent variables

Table 3.4   Production Function Estimates: Disaggregated Physicians (Logarithmic Specification)

Sub-sample	Constant	Beds	Persnl.	Non-labor input	G.P.'s	Surgeons	Med. spec.	Other spec.	Hosp. based	n	$\bar{R}^2$
Full Sample	4.1	.068 (2.1)	.53 (16.1)	.13 (8.1)	.088 (6.1)	.059 (4.9)	.028 (2.1)	.037 (3.4)	−.001 (0.1)	1145	.869
Beds>100	4.3	.14 (3.0)	.45 (9.1)	.11 (3.7)	.049 (2.6)	.080 (3.8)	.034 (2.0)	.038 (2.4)	.033 (3.7)	421	.856
Beds: 50–100	4.1	−.001 (0.2)	.56 (13.0)	.14 (6.9)	.11 (5.6)	.055 (3.7)	.001 (0.2)	.029 (1.9)	−.043 (2.1)	724	.662
Governmental	4.0	−0.0 (0.0)	.56 (11.2)	.16 (5.3)	.10 (4.3)	.071 (3.8)	.032 (0.1)	.003 (0.1)	−.016 (0.8)	615	.810
Not-for-profit	4.1	.13 (3.1)	.47 (10.2)	.12 (8.2)	.082 (4.6)	.046 (2.9)	.025 (1.6)	.078 (5.2)	.012 (0.9)	530	.910
Not-for-profit Beds>100	4.4	.25 (4.0)	.34 (5.8)	.11 (3.2)	.043 (2.1)	.055 (2.0)	.068 (3.4)	.068 (3.4)	.028 (1.6)	240	.888
Not-for-profit Beds 50–100	4.1	.036 (0.0)	.55 (10.0)	.12 (5.0)	.14 (4.7)	.065 (3.3)	−.057 (1.9)	.067 (2.9)	−.019 (0.5)	291	.709
Govt., Beds>100	4.2	.00 (0.0)	.60 (7.5)	.12 (2.0)	.063 (1.6)	.087 (2.6)	.008 (0.1)	.00 (0.0)	.026 (0.9)	181	.800
Govt., Beds 50–100	4.3	−.053 (0.8)	.53 (7.7)	.19 (4.9)	.093 (3.3)	.058 (2.6)	.021 (0.8)	−0.0 (0.0)	−.044 (1.6)	434	.643
Occu. >75%	4.2	.017 (0.3)	.49 (9.1)	.18 (6.1)	.097 (4.7)	.12 (6.0)	−.004 (0.2)	.036 (1.9)	−.005 (0.1)	463	.893

Table 3.5   **Annual Marginal Admission Products, by Physician Specialty Type, Evaluated at Mean**

Subsample	All M.D.'s	G.P.'s	Surg. spec.	Med. spec.	Other spec.	Hosp. based
Full sample	35.8	31.3	46.0	36.7	48.4	——
Beds>100	33.3	21.2	53.5	37.7	44.8	73.2
Beds 50–100	34.8	31.8	54.3	——	——	——
Governmental	32.6	32.3	60.5	48.3	——	——
Not-for-profit	38.9	32.0	32.8	28.9	95.9	——
NFP, Beds>100	34.7	20.6	34.7	68.3	76.1	——
NFP, Beds 50–100	44.1	39.9	62.6	——	98.7	——
Govt. Beds>100	30.1	23.7	63.6	——	——	——
Govt. Beds 50–100	27.9	27.0	56.0	——	——	——
Occu.>75%	38.1	38.0	84.5	——	44.3	——

NOTE: —— = coefficient not significant or negative.

(line 1, table 3.6). While approvals were significant and positively related to admissions (somewhat unexpectedly), their inclusion did not affect the production function coefficients nor contribute appreciably to the explanatory power of the regression. The number of facilities was not significant.

Measuring hospital labor input with the number of full-time-equivalent personnel is obviously imperfect. One possible way to improve the measure of labor input is to follow Feldstein's procedure with British hospitals and use payroll expense. If personnel are heterogeneous, if relative wages reflect relative marginal products, and if absolute wage levels do not differ, the implicit weighting by wage rates should provide a better input measure than does just counting all employees equally. Even though there is no reason to suppose that quality-constant wage levels are identical, the variation among this set of geographically homogeneous hospitals may not be too severe. Line 3 of table 3.6 shows the result of replacing personnel with payroll. In general, using payroll instead of personnel did not improve, and sometimes worsened, the explanatory power of the regression. The only exception is in the case of smaller not-for-profit hospitals. One other change was an increase in the coefficient on beds.

A final test was to change the measure of annual bed cost used in calculating nonlabor expense from $1000 to $3500. Except for the expected change in the relative magnitudes of the *BED* and *NLIP* coefficients, the results were unaffected.

Since it is unclear whether hospital outputs respond immediately to the presence of all inputs, especially beds, medical staff, and specialized

Table 3.6   Alternative Specifications of Production Function: Full Sample

Line	Beds	M.D.'s	Time	Pay-roll	Per-sonnel	NLIP Beds-1000	NLIP Beds-3500	Ap-prov-als	Facil-ities	Avg. Stay	$\bar{R}^2$	n
1.	.064 (2.1)	.15 (10.1)	-.028 (7.8)		.53 (12.0)	.14 (8.7)		.043 (4.1)	-.00 (0.0)		.867	1145
2.	.48 (20.3)	.055 (6.1)	-.027 (11.3)		.34 (14.3)	.11 (10.8)				-.66 (40.2)	.947	1145
3.	.18 (6.2)	.16 (10.5)	-.061 (15.4)	.44 (18.7)		.10 (5.8)					.861	1145
4.	.17 (5.1)	.16 (10.2)	-.026 (7.1)		.55 (16.3)		.030 (7.8)				.863	1145
5.	-.04 (0.1)	.13 (4.1)	—		.69 (7.0)	.11 (2.2)					.906	168

facilities, since the precise dating of when an input was actually available in questionable in the data, and since standard errors may be understated owing to the presence of serial correlation in the pooled time-series cross section, results were also obtained using seven-year average values for each hospital for inputs and outputs. The results are shown on line 5, table 3.6. The results are again very similar to the pooled results of table 3.1, except that the beds variable is now insignificant.

Length of Stay

Holding beds constant, the only ways physician input (or any other input) can increase the number of cases treated are either by increasing the occupancy rate or by reducing length of stay. Feldstein's results for the United Kingdom strongly suggest that when output is increased by increased medical input (or any other input), average duration of stay declines but the occupancy rate is only slightly affected.[8] Does additional physician input in this sample of U.S. hospitals also increase output primarily by shortening stay? One way to tell is by including average stay directly in the production function. One can either interpret this as a "characteristic" of output which one may wish to hold constant, or as another output of a multiproduct firm.[9]

Line 2 of table 3.6 suggests that reductions in stay are an important part of the way in which physicians contribute to output. The coefficient of mean stay is negative and significant; its inclusion substantially improves the $\bar{R}^2$. The coefficient on MD's falls to about one-third of its former value, the coefficients on personnel and $NLIP$ fall by 25–35%, while the coefficient on beds increases substantially. One possible conclusion is indeed that an important way in which physicians "produce" admissions is by shortening the length of stay. It also appears that one of the reasons why the effect of beds on admissions was relatively slight is that beds produce bed-days, and that many of these additional days show up as extended stays rather than as new admissions.

There are, of course, some other explanations which are consistent with these results. One is that there are substantial differences in case complexity, and complexity tends to be positively related to the number of beds and negatively related to the number of physicians.

Another, perhaps more plausible explanation is indicated by Fuchs in his review of Feldstein's book.[10] He suggests that length of stay may vary for reasons other than medical input—regional differences in medical practice, socioeconomic characteristics of patients and area, and so on. If physician input primarily "produces" admissions, not days of stay, while beds and (to a lesser extent) personnel do produce days of stay, a consequence of reduced length of stay will be an increase in the ratio of medical staff to hospital inputs, but the increased ratio does nothing to *cause* the reduction in stay. This explanation would imply that there was, in some sense, an "excess" of days of stay (at least in the sense of their not being needed for the production of a treated case) when medical input was less; it suggests that some hospital inputs cannot be substituted for medical inputs in the production of treated cases. With the available data it is not possible to tell which interpretation is correct.

Optimal Input Ratios

If the hospital were to minimize cost for a given output, it would choose that mix of inputs at which the ratio of regression coefficients (output elasticities) just equalled the ratio of expenditures on the inputs. (This statement assumes that inputs are purchased at constant prices.) For those inputs for which dollar cost estimates are available—personnel, nonlabor inputs, and beds—the optimal ratios and the actual sample mean input expenditure ratios are shown in table 3.7. For physicians, the table shows the shadow price of a physician—the price per physician which would yield an actual ratio of inputs equal to the optimal one. A shadow price for physicians relative to all hospital inputs is also obtained by calculating the price per physician which would produce equality between the ratio of physician costs to hospital costs and the ratio of the coefficient on physicians to the sum of all hospital input coefficients.

There are two main messages from these computations. First, hospitals tend to underuse personnel relative to nonpersonnel inputs—either beds or other nonpersonnel inputs—in all but large nonprofit hospitals. Second, the shadow price of the physicians' annual input into the production of hospital output was in the neighborhood of $17,000 per year. It was higher for not-for-profit hospitals than for governmental hospitals.

There are other costs that should be considered, if only the data were available. To the extent that increased physician input shortens stays, one should add to the opportunity cost of physician input the explicit and implicit costs of home and other nonhospital inputs used to care for the patient during out-of-hospital convalescence, but subtract the opportunity cost of increased "sick time" that may accompany longer stays.

Physicians do not, on average, spend all of their working hours at the hospital. Instead, most physician working hours are spent in their offices, treating and diagnosing ambulatory patients. How does this fact affect the interpretation of the appropriate input mix?

Suppose for the moment that the ratio of average physician office hours to hospital hours is constant across the sample hospitals. If what the physician does in his office has no effect on the demand or supply of admissions, if physicians allocate their time to equate net income per

Table 3.7   Optimal Input Ratios and Shadow Prices of Physician Inputs (Using Estimates of Table 3.1)

Sample	BEDS/MDS		PERS/MDS		NLIP/MDS		BEDS + NLIP MDS		All Hosp IP MDS		PERS NLIP + BEDS	
	Opt. Ratio	Price of M.D.	Opt. Ratio	Price of M.D.	Opt. Ratio	Price of M.D.	Opt. Ratio	Price of M.D.	Opt. Ratio	Price of M.D.	Opt. Ratio	Actual Ratio
Full sample	0.57	107	3.47	148	1.00	283	1.57	219	5.04	170	2.20	1.49
Beds>100	1.00	56	3.06	167	0.88	310	1.88	176	4.94	169	1.63	1.53
Beds 50–100	——		4.08	129	1.15	250	1.15	310	5.23	169	3.53	1.43
Governmental	——		4.07	126	1.21	233	1.21	286	5.29	162	3.35	1.48
Not-for-profit	1.05	56	2.65	194	0.75	374	1.82	189	4.47	191	1.45	1.50
NFP, Beds 50–100	0.54	136	2.94	182	0.71	407	1.24	291	4.18	215	2.38	1.48
NFP, Beds>100	1.75	31	2.31	220	1.00	280	2.75	122	5.06	166	0.84	1.52
Govt. Beds 50–100	——		4.82	107	1.73	172	1.73	212	6.55	136	2.73	1.41
Govt. Beds>100	——		4.13	122	0.73	364	0.73	442	4.87	170	5.64	1.57
Occ.>75%	0.38	143	2.76	177	1.12	241	1.47	221	4.24	192	1.88	1.50

NOTE: —— = coefficient not significant at 0.8 or better.

hour worked at every location, and if prices reflect consumer evaluations, an appropriate measure of the opportunity cost of the time spent
per physician per year in the hospital would be average physician net
income per year times the average fraction that hospital hours are of
total working hours.

Even such measures are not easy to obtain, but the following calculations are probably reasonably accurate. Average physician net income
in nonmetropolitan locations was about $39,000 in 1969. For nonmetro-
politan physicians in 1969 hospital visits were about 25% of total patient visits. If one assumes equal time for hospital or office visits, this
suggests that physicians spend, on average, about one-fourth of the work
time at the hospital. If the average physician "wage" per visit is a legitimate measure of his opportunity cost, that cost is about $9750 per year,
compared to a shadow price of $17,000 per year. The conclusion then
is that there is overuse of hospital inputs relative to physician inputs in
all hospitals taken together, and in all types of hospitals except small
governmental ones. The actual savings from moving to an optimal
physician-hospital input ratio in the average not-for-profit hospital in
the sample would be $144,000, or about 8% of total hospital expenses.
To this should be added the net costs (positive or negative) of convalescence out of the hospital owing to shorter stays. The relatively
greater overuse in not-for-profit hospitals, as compared to governmental
ones, is consistent with the notion that physicians may be able to control
not-for-profit hospitals more effectively than they can control governmental hospitals, which at least have an identified political constituency.

Measures of Physician Input

As described above, the initial measure of physician input was the
number of patient care physicians in the county. The ideal measure of
physician input m_H that we seek could be defined as

$$m_H = h \cdot s \cdot M$$

where M is the number of physicians in the county, s is the hospital's
staff of active physicians as a proportion of the total number of physicians in the county, and h is the average number of hours per week
worked at the hospital by each staff physician. Since m_H is measured by
M, there are several possible sources of error. I will argue that if the
estimates above are in error, they will tend to underestimate physician
productivity, and so tend to underestimate the overuse of hospital inputs.

Even if h, s, and M are uncorrelated, M will measure m_H only with
an error. This raises the possibility of a standard errors-in-variables bias
toward zero. Moreover, if either h or s is correlated with M, the coefficient on M will be a biased measure of m_H.

To adjust for such correlation, two things were done: first, data were obtained on the number of physicians with staff appointments at each of the 160 hospitals in late 1972 from the Social Security Administration's "Provider of Services" data. These data, obtained in the process of Medicare certification, list the number of medical staff appointments of various types. The Social Security Administration's survey also provides some more disaggregated measures of the type of personnel.

Physician staff members were divided into two groups: active staff members, and all other staff members (courtesy, honorary, etc.). A comparison of the results for 1972 using alternatively all county M.D.'s and hospital staff members is shown in table 3.8. The coefficient on physicians is only slightly lower when all county physicians are used than when active staff members are used. When the sample is disaggregated, it becomes apparent that, at least in 1972, there is considerable downward bias in the coefficient estimate for larger hospitals when physician input is measured by the total number of physicians in the county, but there was no bias for smaller hospitals. There does seem to be a little evidence, therefore, that overuse of hospital inputs may be somewhat more severe than indicated above.

Second, it may be hypothesized that physician hospital hours and numbers of physicians relative to hospital inputs might be inversely correlated. At least, with demand held constant, the number of hours worked in total by a physician may decline as the number of physicians increases (either because price declines or because of some pro-rata rationing effects). Moreover, as the number of physicians relative to hospital inputs increases, each physician may spend less time at the hospital. This is another reason to suspect that the estimates in table 3.7 may underestimate the overuse of hospital inputs.

One adjustment that can be made is to estimate the effect of physicians with the physician-population ratio held constant. Physicians may work shorter hours (at the hospital and in total) when they are plentiful relative to the population or, as suggested by Reinhardt, the pace of work may be less hectic. The physician-population ratio in this sense may serve as a proxy for hospital hours per physician. However, when the physician-population ratio (or its log) was entered in the regression, it had a significant coefficient only for the small nonprofit hospitals subsample, and the change there in the coefficient on *MD*'s, while positive, was small.

Conclusion

The empirical results presented in this chapter suggest that, once a patient is hospitalized, there will be some overuse of hospital inputs relative to physician inputs. It would be possible to maintain the pro-

Table 3.8   1972 Production Function Estimates Using Physician Staff and Disaggregated Labor

Line	Personnel	NLXP	Beds (AHA)	M.D.'s	Active Staff M.D.'s	Other Staff M.D.'s	Beds (SSA)	R.N.'s	L.P.N.'s	Other Profs.	Other Personnel	n	$\bar{R}^2$
					FULL SAMPLE								
1.	.57 (6.6)	.20 (3.8)	−.01 (0.1)	.10 (3.2)								160	.908
2.	.55 (6.3)	.20 (4.0)	−.02 (0.3)		.13 (3.8)	.019 (1.3)							.911
3.		.21 (3.6)	−.06 (0.0)		.080 (3.6)	.00 (1.3)		.076 (2.3)	.056 (3.6)	.045 (1.6)	.40 (5.6)		.905
4		.18 (3.6)			.12 (3.3)	.018 (1.4)	.19 (2.8)	.040 (1.2)	.046 (2.9)	.045 (1.7)	.32 (5.7)		.915
					BEDS: 50–100								
1.	.55 (5.1)	.21 (3.3)	−.09 (1.0)	.088 (2.1)								101	.792
2.	.55 (4.9)	.22 (3.4)	−.10 (1.1)		.084 (1.9)	−.00 (0.0)							.788
3.		.21 (3.3)	−.06 (0.8)		.808 (1.7)	.00 (0.0)		.092 (1.9)	.059 (2.7)	.035 (0.9)	.38 (4.2)		.786
4.		.21 (3.4)			.076 (1.7)	.00 (0.0)	.12 (1.4)	.058 (1.1)	.051 (2.8)	.032 (0.9)	.30 (4.1)		.789

Table 3.8—*continued*

Line	Personnel	NLXP	Beds (AHA)	M.D.'s	Active Staff M.D.'s	Other Staff M.D.'s	Beds (SSA)	R.N.'s	L.P.N.'s	Other Profs.	Other Personnel	n	$\bar{R}^2$
					BEDS>100								
1.	.50 (3.3)	.27 (2.7)	.11 (1.0)	.066 (1.2)								59	.892
2.	.50 (3.3)	.16 (1.6)	.08 (0.6)		.22 (3.2)	.045 (2.1)							.913
3.		.16 (1.7)	.09 (0.7)		.23 (3.2)	.047 (2.1)		.038 (0.8)	.038 (1.6)	.031 (0.7)	.37 (3.1)		.908
4.		.13 (1.3)			.21 (3.2)	.043 (2.2)	.27 (2.7)	.019 (0.4)	.031 (1.4)	.042 (1.1)	.32 (3.7)		.919

duction of hospital admissions, even while reducing the level of hospital inputs, if additional physicians' time were added. The reduction in cost of the hospital inputs thus saved would *exceed* the increase in costs attributable to the additional physician inputs, at least if the social costs are measured by the portion of physician net income coming from time spent at the hospital. Whether these costs equal the social costs of providing physician services is, of course, very uncertain, given the way in which physician training is financed. Nevertheless, if these output elasticities are accepted as measures of the effect of physician hospital hours, and if the cost measure is taken as appropriate, the conclusion is that the given stock of physicians could be used more efficiently if physicians spent more time at the hospital and hospitals eliminated some personnel and nonlabor inputs.

This is inefficiency in the direction opposite from that found by Reinhardt for office practices. However, it is by no means obvious that a shift toward more physician-intensive production of hospital care would raise physician utility, even though it would lower hospital and total costs. Reductions in hospital costs reduce hospital insurance benefits. Depending upon the amount and type of physician fee insurance, the result may be a decrease in physician utility. Here, at least, we have a *reason* why resource misallocation occurs.

One message for policy is that what is likely to be important is the relatively low marginal product of specialists, especially of surgeons. Given the high cost of training surgeons, one may wonder whether the hospital output, even if that output is thought to be appropriate in some sense, justifies those costs. Of course, in practice, increases in physicians are likely to be accompanied by increases in hospital inputs; the hospital inputs mean more output, but also more cost.

Another message is that even primary care physicians—G.P.'s and medical specialists—have a significant positive effect on hospital admissions. If the goal is to increase the number of primary care physicians *without* increasing the hospitalization rate, the analysis above suggests that an appropriate strategy is to couple physician increases with hospital input decreases.

4   Physician Information and the Consumer's Demand for Care

In chapter 1, I developed the rudiments of a simple model of a consumer's demand for medical care, conditional on the level of health physicians had led him to expect to result. In this chapter, I shall examine in much more detail how consumer expectations are formed.

If consumers always believed all that physicians told them, and accepted advice unquestioningly, then the only constraint on movement to that level of demand which would maximize physician income—probably a very high level of demand indeed—would be the moral scrupulousness of physicians. The physician's attitude toward truth-telling, or "accuracy" as I shall call it hereafter, can be shown to be an important influence on a consumer's use of care and on health levels, but it may not be the only influence. In particular, consumers can control the effect of physician-provided information on their behavior by deciding, within some limits, both how to react to advice and which physicians to patronize for advice. In some emergencies, the consumer does not of course have these options. But the bulk of medical encounters are not of this sort, and even in many situations labeled "emergency" the consumer has in principle a considerable amount of power over what can be done to him (including whether or not he chooses to be an "emergency" case) and which physician he chooses in order to obtain advice.

In view of recent questioning of the appropriateness of medical advice and medical decisions from such diverse parties as Ivan Illich[1] and the U.S. House of Representatives Subcommittee on Oversight and Investigations,[2] it seems appropriate to determine whether a more analytical approach to the question can make a contribution. As will soon become apparent, even a designedly simple approach to modeling the problem soon becomes quite complicated.

43

What will determine how a consumer will react to physician advice? Intuitively, one might suppose that the stronger a person's prior beliefs, the less he will respond to the information provided. Unfortunately, this conjecture is incorrect in general for reasonable measures of "strength of beliefs." But it is still possible to show that for some sufficiently high level of prior certainty, this conclusion will follow. Thus there is a theoretical basis for the empirical expectation that those spending units characterized by a sufficiently high level of a priori information will, other things being equal, be less responsive to changes in information obtained.

The model is one in which the consumer's demand for medical care is conditional on the content of the advice. There are two critical questions to be addressed: (1) What determines from which physician he will seek advice? (2) What determines how the consumer will respond to the advice? Corresponding to each of these aspects of demand, there is an appropriate supply response: first, the content of the advice each physician decides to provide; and second, the overall content of advice physicians choose. In what follows I will examine each of these decisions.

The Consumer's Demand for Medical Care

The approach here is first to develop a simple model of the consumer's demand for medical care under certainty, then introduce uncertainty but with information unavailable, and finally to show the consequences of permitting information to become available. One possible aspect of behavior that will not be incorporated here is a possible consumer suspicion, based solely on the content of the advice received, that the physician is willfully not providing accurate information. In the model to be discussed, the physician may lie, and the consumer may not believe him, but consumers do not believe that physicians individually or collectively lie on purpose; physicians are only supposed to make honest mistakes.

It is assumed that the consumer has a single period utility function in health H and other goods x. The intertemporal aspects of the choice of health levels and of the production process for health, which have been treated extensively by Grossman,[3] will be ignored here. Likewise the time cost of obtaining health will be ignored. As in chapter 1, the utility function is

(1) $$U = U(x, H)$$

The composite good x is available at a price of unity, but health must be produced. The production function for health is

(2) $$H = g(M, H_o)$$

The marginal health product of medical care g_1 is positive, the effect on final health of H_o (or g_2) is positive, and g_1 is larger the smaller the value of H_o, or $g_{12} < 0$ (i.e., medical care benefits people more the sicker they are). For simplicity, it is assumed that, given H_o, g_1 is a constant, i.e., there is a constant marginal and average health product. If the consumer knows with certainty that the value of H_o is $\bar{H}_o$ and the value of g_1 for that H_o is $\bar{g}_1$, then his problem is to maximize (1) subject to

(2') $$H = \bar{H}_o + \bar{g}_1 \cdot M$$

and

(3) $$Y = x + pM.$$

Given his endowment (Y, H_o) and the shadow price of health, g_1/p, the consumer chooses the amount of health he wishes to buy.

The consumer might be uncertain either because he does not know H_o or because he does not know g_1 for a given H_o. That is, he might be uncertain either about what is wrong with him, which determines H_o, or how effective medical care is in dealing with his condition, which determines g_1. (In a more complex but realistic model, g_1 might depend not just upon H_o, but upon the particular disease the person has. But for simplicity I will continue to assume that conditions are only classified by severity.)

The first case to be considered is that in which g_1 is uncertain but H_o is known. Suppose g_1 (given H_o) has the (subjective) distribution $f(g_1)$. The problem then is to maximize expected utility:

(4) $$EU = \int U(x - pM, H_o + g_1 M) f(g_1) \, dg_1$$

subject to constraint (3). Solution of this problem implies that M is chosen so that $\pi_i u'(g^i_1) = \pi_j u'(g^j_1)$, where π_i and π_j are the probabilities attached to two alternate values of g_1. In effect, the consumer chooses a level of M that would be somewhat appropriate for all possible states, but ideally appropriate for almost none.

Now assume that the consumer can obtain information on H_o or g_1 from the physician. In order to explain how the consumer will respond to any given information, it is necessary to explain how he judges the accuracy (or diagnostic and prescriptive skill) of a physician. One way the consumer can tell whether a physician is giving him accurate advice is to observe the results of experiments. Those experiments would take the following form: suppose g_1 is uncertain but H_o is known. Suppose a physician asserts that the value of g_1 is $\bar{g}_1$. The consumer would then observe whether $H = H_o + \bar{g}_1 \bar{M}$ when he uses $\bar{M}$ units of care.

The result of a single such experiment will ordinarily not be conclusive. H might differ from $H_o + \bar{g}_1 \bar{M}$ for a number of reasons. For example, the true production process might be $H = H_o + g_1 M + u$, $E(u) = 0$, $\sigma^2_u > 0$. Then additional observations on sample values of g_1 would be needed to get an estimate of the population mean of (actual) g_1. Given some a priori distribution, the consumer can make an estimate of the accuracy with which this physician predicts g_1. A similar argument holds for H_o. Note that the physician's motivation is irrelevant here.

Suppose then a person is trying to determine whether or not he would buy diagnostic information, and from which physician he would purchase it. His "information about the accuracy of the information" will be relevant. What will determine the amount of such information he possesses? It is the number of experiments he has observed, or the price of additional experiments. These "experiments" will represent his own encounters with the physician, or those of his friends. Moreover, his own skill in evaluating observed results may also affect his perceptions of informational accuracy. Given his own and others' experiences, the consumer can come to subjective estimates of the value of g_1, and of the accuracy of physician conjectures about the level of g_1.

Now consider the effect of such estimates on the consumer's choices. Suppose g^τ_1 is the actual value of g_1. Suppose the physician can determine g^τ_1. Finally, suppose the person is given information by a physician on what the value of g_1 is; this physician advice is represented by g^ϕ_1, and is not necessarily equal to g^τ_1. If the person's prior distribution were $f(g_1)$, his posterior distribution $f(g_1|g^\phi_1)$ is given by Bayes' rule as

$$f(g_1|g^\phi_1) = \frac{f(g^\phi_1|g_1)}{f(g^\phi_1)} \cdot f(g_1)$$

where

$$f(g^\phi_1) = \int f(g^\phi_1|g_1)\, f(g_1)$$

In each case, the value of $f(g_1)$ is adjusted by the ratio of the conditional to the unconditional distribution of $f(g^\phi_1)$. We can immediately distinguish two special cases. First, suppose the person knows the truth with certainty. Consequently, the prior and posterior distributions are the same. Information does not affect this person's demand for care at all.

The alternative case is one in which the person puts complete confidence in the physician's opinion, so that his posterior estimate of g_1 is identical to what the physician tells him.

If physicians tell the truth ($g^\phi_1 = g^\tau_1$), then M will be set at M_τ for both kinds of persons. If physicians are not always accurate, then the person who is certain of the truth still chooses M_τ, but the person who believes the physician will choose some quantity other than M_τ. If persons are of either of these two extreme types, an empirical measure that distinguishes them permits one to make predictions about the possible responsiveness of demand to physician information which has varying degrees of accuracy.

Difficulties arise when either the a priori distribution or the likelihood function are not of the degenerate forms discussed here. While it is easy to show that the change in probability π attached to same value of g_1 in response to information, given some likelihood function, is smaller the larger is $|\pi - 1/2|$, it does not follow that the change in the preferred level of M will be smaller. That depends on how the preferred M changes with changes in π. If M changes very rapidly with changes in π for a π in excess of $1/2$, then it is possible that information may make a bigger difference in the use of such persons as compared to the use of more "uncertain" persons, with π closer to $1/2$. One can say that the response to new information of the individual's use of care is likely to be different for persons with different prior beliefs or prior stocks of information. But it does not appear that one can make any general a priori conjectures about the direction of this relationship.

However, theoretical determinateness can be salvaged if the extremes are considered. It can be said that one can find some π sufficiently close to 1 or zero that the effect on preferred M of the message $g_1 = g^{\phi}_1$ is smaller than the effect of that message on use at any π further away from these extremes. Since the effect of any change in π on M must be finite, if we can find some $\Delta\pi$ (as a result of receiving information) that is sufficiently small, we can get as small an effect on M as we want. All we need to show is that, in the neighborhood of $\pi = 1$, we can find a π such that $\Delta\pi$ as a result of the message $g_1 = g^{\phi}_1$ is as small as we want. Consider some value of $\pi = (1 - \epsilon)$. Since the physician's advice has no effect when $\pi = 1$, by continuity it follows that, by selecting some value of ϵ sufficiently small, we can make $f(g_1|g^{\phi}_1 \neq g^{\tau}_1)$ as close to $f(g_1)$ as we want for any given likelihood function.[4] That is, we can make the posterior probability as close to the prior probability as we want, even if the physician provides incorrect information.

This discussion of the effect of information on use suggests that, however indeterminate the relationship in general, one can find sufficiently extreme values of information and ignorance such that the informed are less responsive to information than the ignorant. This proposition will be the basis of the empirical analysis.

A Censoring Problem

This proposition applies only if the set of conditions for which informed and uninformed persons receive physician advice is the same. Such an assumption may not be plausible in general. One problem is that the incidence of conditions may differ according to the level of information, but this problem is not likely to be serious. A more serious problem arises from a kind of censoring. The person who is virtually certain of the truth will ignore erroneous physician advice, as described in the preceding section. But he will also have no incentive to seek that advice in the first place. Those persons in the "well-informed" set who actually meet with physicians will tend to be precisely those whose behavior is easier to change; the unresponsive persons will have been "censored" out initially, independent of the eventual content of physician advice. Those persons classified as poorly informed who seek advice may therefore be no more responsive than those persons classified as well informed who seek advice.

This difficulty will not be important if persons who seek medical therapy usually must first see a physician and get his advice (or at least his diagnosis), whether they demand that advice or not. Suppose, for example, a child in a well-informed family has tonsilitis. The parents know that tonsillectomy is not warranted for his condition. Nevertheless, they must go through a physician in order to obtain a prescription for antibiotics, and are therefore potentially exposed to the content of physician advice.

It seems reasonable to suppose that many conditions for which demand creation is likely are of this sort; at least one physician contact is often needed for therapy, no matter what the state of patient information. As long as those persons in the well-informed set who really do seek advice (i.e., are not virtually certain) are not *more* responsive than those in the less well-informed set, the elasticity, and probably the magnitude, of the response of the well-informed who use positive amounts of care will be smaller than that of the less well-informed. This occurs because the well-informed set will include some persons who really are virtually certain, but are compelled to go through at least one physician in order to obtain any care at all. That is, as long as some of those persons who are truly well-informed are persons who seek care (even if they do not seek advice), the overall response of persons in the well-informed set will be smaller, other things being equal.

The Level of Accuracy, the Demand for Care, and Physician Availability

The empirical finding for which we seek a theoretical framework is that, *ceteris paribus*, the demand curve for physicians' services appears to shift when the stock of physicians per capita changes, because accuracy of physician advice decreases. The purpose of this section is to construct models which are consistent with a negative relationship between physicians per capita and accuracy. It is not my intent to argue that a negative relationship *must* hold. A model is useful if it *permits* a negative relationship to hold; as will be shown, certain otherwise attractive and plausible models do not permit a negative relationship to occur, and so those models must be discarded.

For the purpose of distinguishing among models, the classification in chapter 1 is useful. To begin with, there is no point in discussing competitive market clearing models. If the seller takes price as given and supposes that he can sell as much as he wants at that price, there is no reason for him to alter accuracy in order to sell more. Consequently, the discussion will primarily be concerned with noncompetitive models.

Model 1: The Physician as a Real-income Maximizing Monopolist

The usual assumption in studies of labor supply is that the agents have two arguments in their utility functions: money income and leisure. In order to simplify the exposition, it will be assumed that physician time is available at a constant opportunity cost. This assumption avoids the necessity of including leisure in the utility function, and makes maximization of utility equivalent to maximization of the difference between total revenue and total opportunity costs, including the opportunity cost of leisure foregone.

The physician may be thought of as selling two products: diagnostic information and therapeutic care. These markets are not separate. The amount of information about a product that consumers will want to buy will depend upon both the price of information *and* the price of the product, in this case therapeutic care. Likewise, the amount of therapeutic care that a person will eventually buy at a given price will depend upon the price of information. Although the quantity of each type of care demanded is inversely related to its own price, it is not possible to establish definitive comparative statics results for the cross-price effects. The problem is further complicated in practice by the nonmarginal nature of many information purchases. Often in order to receive any therapeutic care at all the individual is required to seek diagnosis; in principle the price of diagnostic information could absorb all of the consumers' surplus from therapeutic care.

But the concern here is not primarily with these price and quantity effects. Rather, we wish to determine the accuracy or the content of a *given* amount of information purchased. Assume initially that the accuracy of the diagnosis does not affect a physician's information demand curve. Holding other things constant, including leisure time and the physician time devoted to diagnosis and therapeutic care, the real-income maximizing physician will then adjust the level of accuracy A to that level at which the increase in his net income from changing accuracy is zero. This conclusion implies that, for any quantity of therapeutic care demanded, accuracy is set at that level which maximizes the unit price paid.

If total demand for therapeutic care Q_D is given by $Q_D = Q(P, A)$, where P is the user price of care and A is the level of accuracy among a set of identical physicians, then the individual physician demand Q^i_D, assuming pro-rata sharing among N identical physicians, is $Q^i_D = 1/N \, Q_D(P, A)$. The individual physician demand curve when A is set at the level of true information, or A_T, is shown in figure 4.1 as $D^i_T = 1/N \, Q_D(P, A_T)$. But the maximizing physician will not choose to confront this curve; instead he will probably choose that level of accuracy which

Price

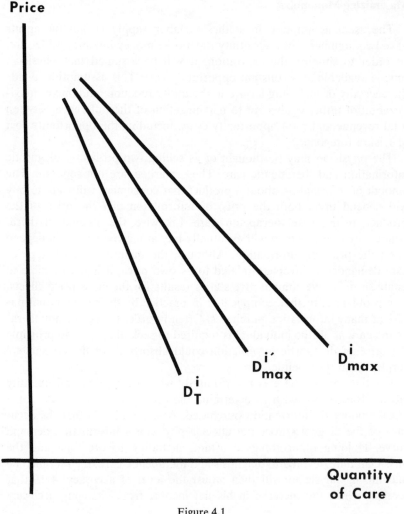

Figure 4.1

maximizes price at every quantity. This choice yields a maximum curve, $D^i_{max} = 1/N \, Q_D(P, A_{max})$, where A_{max} is the level of accuracy which maximizes P at every Q_D. He will then choose the profit-maximizing level of P given this curve.

The effect of increasing the supply of physicians can be thought of as a pro-rata decrease in the demand facing each physician. (It might also change the extent of competitiveness, but that will be ignored here.) The D^i_{max} curve will shift to $D^{i\prime}_{max}$, the result being smaller output per physician at any price, and probably a lower price. However, this change will not necessarily affect the level of accuracy, and it will have no effect on the market demand curve D^i_{max}. That level of accuracy which maximizes price at a given quantity demanded from a particular seller also maximizes price at any pro-rata share of that quantity. There would, in this situation, be *no* detectable availability effect resulting from an increase in the number of physicians (even though demand is, of course, different from D_T). Quantity demanded would rise as price falls along the D^i_{max} demand curve, but this would be wholly captured in an accurate measure of user price. Any observed availability effect must be due to changes in nonmonetary rationing. If we are to postulate a measurable availability effect arising from information, we must enlarge the set of arguments in the physician's utility function.

Model 2: The Physician as a Partially Benevolent Oligopolist

In this section we shall consider a model of demand creation among physicians who take price as given but do not expect to be able to sell unlimited amounts at that price. In addition to being realistic, especially for situations in which third parties set fee levels, this model permits us to throw into sharp focus the physician's incentive to alter accuracy.

It may not be unreasonable to assume that alterations in accuracy operate mainly on quantity, not price, at least as far as the individual physician is concerned. Oligopolistic features of the industry may lead to a reluctance to raise price, as may a kind of altruism that recognizes that higher prices give no benefit to consumers, while higher quantities may provide some benefit to both consumers and physicians.

It is assumed that physicians are partially benevolent, in the sense that the physician's maximand also includes a measure of accuracy. Other things being equal, physicians would rather tell the truth, but they would be willing to surrender some accuracy for some amount of money income. The physician obtains utility from real income Y, which is total revenue minus total opportunity costs, and from accuracy A. Both real income and accuracy are normal goods.

With P fixed, the physician who does not get utility from accuracy will choose that level of accuracy at which the quantity demanded from him equals or gets as close as possible (given demand) to that quantity at which price equals "marginal cost," where the latter includes the value of sacrificed leisure. However, when accuracy yields utility, the level of accuracy is the one which satisfies

(5) $$\frac{U_A}{U_Y} = (P - \partial C/\partial Q) \; \partial Q/\partial A$$

where C is total opportunity cost, including the opportunity cost of physician time, and U_A and U_Y are the marginal utilities of accuracy and income respectively.

These effects are shown in figure 4.2. Suppose price is initially at P, and "MC" measures both money marginal cost and the money value of sacrificed leisure. At any P, income would obviously be maximized by setting Q either at that Q at which $P = $ "MC" or at the Q on the D^i_{max}

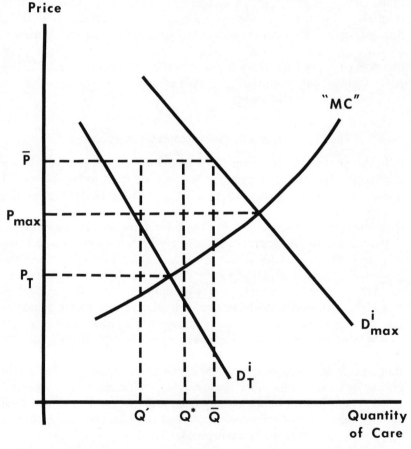

Figure 4.2

demand curve, whichever is less. If $P = \bar{P}$, for example, Q would be set at $\bar{Q}$. But if the physician values accuracy, he may not be willing to expand Q (and reduce A) to this level. He may instead set accuracy at the level given by equation (5), and consequently set Q at, say, Q^* less than $\bar{Q}$.

Now let the number of physicians be increased. Each physician's Q will fall below Q^*, say to Q', if A stays at its initial level. At this point, the physician's income is less so he may be willing to sacrifice some accuracy to recoup part of the loss in income. (Ordinarily he would not wish to reduce accuracy so much as to restore his original level of income.) Moreover, at Q', there will also be a bigger gain from increasing Q by one unit, since $P - \text{``}MC\text{''}$ is greater. If $\partial Q / \partial A$ is constant or increases as Q decreases, then the net return from changing A will also have increased.

As with most oligopoly models, this model does not make specific predictions about the equilibrium level of price. It is likely that price would decline below $\bar{P}$, though by how much, and to what extent the decline would be related to physicians per capita, is impossible to say. But whatever the final price, at that price there would generally be some incentive to create demand. Moreover, the incentive to create demand would generally be greater at a given price the larger the number of physicians.

There would, however, be no incentive to create demand if the price settled to P_T or below. Note that if P equals P_T, a physician, even an income-maximizing one, would tell the truth; an incentive to create demand requires excess supply at P_T. This is an important result, and it will be discussed in more detail later in this chapter. Note also that P_T falls as physician stock increases.

If price is given but is initially below P_{max}, then use will increase with physician stock *even if* physicians only value income, not accuracy. In effect, use is constrained by supply, and follows the outward-shifting aggregate supply curve. The more elastic supply is, the less likely that price is below P_{max}. For example, if there are constant returns to scale in the supply of some type of physician service, the quantity given by the D_{max} demand curve will be supplied for any price in excess of average cost, and no availability effect will be observed.

Figure 4.2 also indicates that, *given* the number of physicians, the extent of demand creation will vary positively with the price, unless income effects are very strong. The reward from creating demand, or $P - MC$, is obviously larger at any Q the higher P is. Of course, income will also be higher if P is higher, and this "income effect" may to some extent offset the "substitution effect" in the direction of reduced accuracy.

Model 3: The Physician as a Partially Benevolent Monopolist

If the physician has some control over price, it is still true that in equilibrium the marginal effect of changes in accuracy on his income must compensate him for the disutility of reduced accuracy. The effect that changes in accuracy have on the level of income depends upon *how* the demand curve is shifted when A changes. Whatever price is finally charged, the marginal condition (5) must obviously still be satisfied. In addition, the usual $MR = MC$ condition, given the level of accuracy, must hold as well. By the same arguments as in the preceding section, the level of accuracy will decrease with the physician stock at any *given* level of price if $\partial Q / \partial A$ is constant or increases with decreases in Q. Consequently, one would expect to observe an availability effect on consumer demands.

This appears to be the only unambiguous prediction one can obtain from "demand-creation" models. As Feldman and Sloan[5] have shown, and as Reinhardt[6] has emphasized, literally any relationship between equilibrium market price and physician stock is consistent with such models. Depending upon how the demand curve pivots when it shifts, the new equilibrium price could be above, equal, or below the price that prevailed with a smaller stock of physicians.

This result has led both Evans[7] and Reinhardt to conclude that it is not possible to refute the demand creation hypothesis by looking at the relationship between physician stock and price. The most that such an investigation could do is to cast doubts on the neoclassical competitive hypothesis of no demand creation. Even this weak conclusion is really not very useful. If the market is monopolistic rather than competitive, and individual physician demand curves become less elastic as the physician stock rises, then price can vary directly with that stock even in a neoclassical, income-maximizing, but noncompetitive world. While one usually does not assume that firm demand curves become less elastic when more competitors enter, Satterthwaite[8] has recently shown that the effect of numbers of sellers on information about prices or quality levels of providers can lead to such a result without having consumers pushed off their "true" demand curve by changes in accuracy. Moreover, Pauly and Satterthwaite[9] have found that variation in the level of prices across cities can be explained without recourse to the modified target income model.

The relationship between price and availability will therefore not settle the question of the availability effect, but a study of the relationship between availability and use, *given* price, and between price and use, *given* availability, will provide some answers. These answers will be valid even if prices are not fixed, as long as price is exogenous to the individual demander. It is precisely this kind of test that will be presented in the next chapter.

Information about Information

Up to this point, we have taken the consumer's estimate of the accuracy of physician advice as depending only on the total number of experiments or experiences he has observed. We have also assumed that the consumer does not change physicians in response to the content of information provided by the physician; the consumer's only decision is whether to follow that advice or not. But consumers may well perceive differences among physicians with regard to the accuracy of their advice, and act on those perceptions in choosing which physician to patronize. In other words, the individual physician firm's demand curves for its output of advice and for its output of therapeutic care may increase if it is perceived to give more accurate advice. Such a response may provide an incentive to the physician to offer accurate advice; it constrains his ability to generate net increases in demand. In terms of the geometric presentation, competition may affect the position of the D^i_{max} curve; whether or not it actually pushes the curve in as far as D^i_T, competition may still affect the observed level of accuracy.

We now need to ask how competition, as measured by the number of physicians (in total or per capita), affects the equilibrium level of accuracy. While a complete characterization of this kind of equilibrium with information and goods as joint products has not yet been fully developed, the following simple model possesses what appear to be critical insights.

Suppose a market area has N identical patients (customers) and M identical physicians (sellers). Suppose that the selling price of therapeutic care is fixed at $\bar{P}$, which is above "MC" at the output of therapeutic care demanded when the truth is told. Suppose profits are only earned on therapeutic care. At any level of accuracy A, let demand per patient be $Q(A)$; demand per physician is $\frac{NQ}{M}$. Suppose that each physician takes other physicians' levels of accuracy as given. Finally, suppose that any one physician expects that, if all other physicians maintain their (identical) levels of accuracy, and he raises his, he will obtain some fraction k of all other physicians' customers.

Given some initial level of accuracy, a physician's income will then be increased by increases in his level of accuracy if

$$k \cdot \frac{NQ}{M} \cdot (M-1) > \frac{\partial Q}{\partial A} \frac{N}{M}$$

The term on the left is the gain to the physician of k percent of the $\left(\dfrac{NQ}{M}\right)$ services provided by each of the $M - 1$ other physicians. The term on the right is the loss to the physician resulting from less demand among his current set of customers. Simplification of the inequality indicates that an increase in accuracy will increase income if $kQ\,(M - 1) > \partial Q/\partial A$.

If k and $\partial Q/\partial A$ are assumed to be constant, the expression obviously implies that accuracy will tend to increase as the number of physicians (or competitors) increases. But while there is no obvious reason why $\partial Q/\partial A$ should change as M changes, there are some reasons why k might vary with M. On the one hand, standard search models would suggest that, if accuracy can be measured with certainty by just one search, k would be likely to increase with M. The more sellers, the lower the average cost to the consumer of getting an "accuracy quotation" from another seller, and consequently the more attractive will be a higher accuracy seller. There is a second possibility, however, if the level of accuracy is not measured perfectly. Given some total number of experiments or experiences, the consumer's estimate of the accuracy of a *particular* physician's diagnosis will be likely to depend on the total number of physicians in his market area. The more physicians, the lower the average number of experiences the consumer or his friends are likely to have had with any given physician, and hence the less precisely he can estimate the quality or accuracy of any individual physician's diagnosis. If there is only one physician in town, all of the consumer's past experience will have been with that physician. If there are hundreds of physicians, the *average* accuracy of his estimate will be less (although he could have a very accurate estimate of the diagnostic capability of any individual physician). If the consumer is risk averse, or if he has difficulty remembering the identities of multiple sellers, he may be less willing to leave his present seller (whose accuracy he probably knows fairly well) for another physician whose accuracy he can estimate only imperfectly. To take two extremes: in a town with only a few physicians, differential levels of accuracy will quickly become well known. But in a large metropolitan area, it may be very difficult to find several friends who use the same physician, so that it will be impossible to get an accurate measure of the level of accuracy of any alternative seller. Consequently, it is possible that k will tend to be larger in small towns than in large metropolitan areas; k may well decrease as the number of physicians increases.

An availability effect will be nonexistent, or small and difficult to detect, if D_{max} is close to D_T. What do the observations above imply about measurement of the availability effect? They suggest that the position of the D_{max} demand curve is likely to vary with the number of physicians (*not* physicians per capita) in the market area. The relationship between number of physicians and D_{max} cannot, however, be predicted a priori: D_{max} can increase, decrease, or remain constant as M changes. The relationship depends upon the sign and magnitude of the rate of change in k with respect to M. Moreover, precise measurement of the extent of market area is probably impossible, although there have been some fairly successful attempts to use proxy measures.[10] It does seem possible, nevertheless, to characterize extreme cases. In rural areas, at one extreme, the level of consumer information is likely to be fairly high, so it is possible that D_{max} will be fairly close to D_T—little or no availability effect will be observed, because it will not pay physicians to reduce their level of accuracy when some consumers are able to detect the reduction.[11] In large metropolitan areas, at the other extreme, it is likely that k will be low, possibly near zero, because few of the consumer's friends are likely to be able to provide information on the same physician's accuracy. Consequently, D_{max} will lie far to the right of D_T, and the "standard" availability effect analysis developed above will apply.

While these statements are obviously highly conjectural, they do suggest that, in the absence of accurate measures of the number of sellers in the consumers' market area, it may be desirable to estimate separate availability effects for rural areas, large metropolitan areas, and other areas. Such a procedure is followed in the empirical work described in the next chapter.

Incentives Under a Fee-for-service System

Before going on to discuss the outcomes produced by the physician incentives present in the existing fee-for-service system, I will digress to examine fee-for-service under alternative fee schedules. The goal here is to see whether there is something inherent in the fee-for-service concept which leads to departures from accurate advice. One of the results from the analysis earlier in this chapter that deserves special emphasis is the following: if the physician's notional supply curve intersects that consumer's demand curve which corresponds to true and accurate information, then the price at which this intersection occurs is a price which will induce the physician to tell the truth, and act as the consumer's agent. In this section I wish to expand on this notion, to extend it to a model in which there are multiple kinds of outputs supplied by the physician, and to use it to analyze the possible superiority of prepaid group practice or Health Maintenance Organizations (HMOs) over fee-for-service medicine.

With respect to the choice among competing methods of treating a given illness, it is often argued that the fee-for-service physician has an incentive *not* to provide true information and *not* to recommend to the patient the utility-maximizing course of treatment. In particular, the fee-for-service physician, it is argued, will provide too much care as well as unnecessarily expensive forms of care.[12] I explored the issues of cost-minimization for a given level of health in chapter 1, and I argued that (1) the income-maximizing physician may give distorted advice on the level of health to be achieved and (2) if fees are not free to vary, the mix of treatments may not be the one which minimizes the cost of whatever level of health is produced. Here I shall examine the possibility of choosing a schedule of fees to minimize both kinds of distortion.

With respect to fee-for-service versus HMOs, there has been much discussion of the apparent fact that the fee-for-service system of payment tends to encourage additional use of medical care, especially hospitalization, as compared to capitation-salary schemes. Often this finding is extended to a comparison of fee-for-service in general with capitation in general, and often, too, it is argued that the additional use is unnecessary in some normative sense. What I wish to suggest here, however, is that these characteristics of the present fee-for-service system are not, in themselves, evidence against the concept of paying for medical care (or any other good) on a fee-for-service basis. If there are failings in the present system, they may stem *not* from the fee-for-service system as such, but primarily from the present level of actual fees. A possible misallocation of manpower is a secondary (and related) cause. It is not fee-for-service as a concept that is faulty, but rather some changeable characteristics of the present fee-for-service system. It is therefore wrong-headed to argue for a general preference for capitation or salary as opposed to fee-for-service.

In fact, it is possible to establish a stronger result: not only can fee-for-service be made as "good" as capitation, from a theoretical viewpoint, it can be better than any feasible form of capitation. Put another way, there exists some set of fees for specific services which will achieve a pattern of incentives for physicians that, at worst, provides him no incentive to depart from an agency role. Any preference for patient welfare, however slight, would then be sufficient to cause him to act as a perfect agent. These theoretical considerations do not, of course, bear directly on the question of the merits of existing systems, since each may be at different places in the best-worst continuum. They do suggest, however, that even if the present fee-for-service system is not perfect, it is at least perfectible. Accordingly, I shall go on to consider (1) why the present system might not have achieved the ideal pattern of fees and (2) what alterations might improve matters.

Initially, I will assume that the prices (fees) received by physicians are given. This assumption is useful analytically, and may not be too unrealistic when third party payers are involved. Suppose that the total hours physicians will work is given, and suppose physician utility depends on income received and patient well-being. (Physicians do not prefer to do some tasks more than others.) The concern for patient well-being can be very small, in the sense that the physician would be willing to sacrifice a great deal of patient well-being for a very small increase in income. All that is required is that, given a set of actions which yields equal money income, the physician will choose that course of action which most benefits his patients. The question now is: What is the set of prices for individual services the physician prescribes which will cause him to behave in a way which maximizes patient welfare?

The intuitive basis for the answer to this question is clear: if the physician makes the same amount of income no matter how he spends his time with patients, he might as well choose the way which most benefits his patients. That is, a set of prices which equalizes physician net income per hour worked will permit physician utility maximization and patient welfare maximization to coincide.[13]

There is still the question of how total physician hours worked are determined. If physician utility depends on income and leisure, and the other usual conditions are satisfied, then there will be a supply curve of total hours worked for each physician. Given the number of physicians in practice, there will be some overall level of net income per hour worked which will maximize patient welfare.

Contrast the pattern of output which physicians would want to supply under this scheme with that under a scheme in which net income per hour is not equalized. The income-maximizing physician will choose to produce that type of output which yields the highest returns per hour worked. If there were no other constraints, this would be the only type of output he would produce. But there may be limits on the amount of this type of output he can persuade people to take. Then he may produce the next most profitable output, or he may even produce some complementary lower-yield outputs (e.g., initial office visits) in order to be able to persuade consumers to take the higher yield output.

If the production process for each output displays constant returns to scale, then the level of net income from any output will depend on the price of output and the price of inputs, but not on the particular amount of output. If there are increasing costs for a given output, price can be used to select any particular quantity or mix of output. In the first case, the most that can be accomplished is what might be called "incentive neutrality": the physician would be indifferent toward producing the ideal mix of output and some other combination of those outputs which are to be produced in positive quantities. However, if the physician has the slightest preference for doing what is in the patient's best interest, or if there is the slightest chance that he will lose patients in whose interests he does not act, then he will behave as a perfect agent. In the second case, the total quantity of each type of output produced by each physician is determined by the price, but not the mix provided to each patient. Again, a slight degree of concern for patient welfare or a slight extent of competition is all that is needed for the optimal outcome to be an equilibrium outcome.

Compare these ideal price incentives to those under a capitation (HMO) system. Total revenue is fixed, so real income maximization provides incentives to minimize total inputs, whether physician or nonphysician. For the income-maximizing (or cost-minimizing HMO), there are incentives to provide a small amount of total output, even when that would not be in the patient's own interests, and to select cheaper mixes of outputs. Competition may constrain the ability to underprovide somewhat, but it is unlikely that it will be perfect enough to prevent it entirely. This is not to say that an HMO equilibrium may not be preferable to existing fee-for-service prices. However, there exists a set of fee-for-service prices, not necessarily existing ones, which can always do as well or better, in terms of providing incentives for agency, than any capitation scheme. For a capitation scheme to achieve even as good an outcome as fee-for-service, perfect competition is required. Perfect competition is *not* required under the ideal set of fees-for-service.[14]

Comparisons between existing fee-for-service and HMO systems are made difficult because of an ambiguity in the notion of agency, which has been noted above. With insurance that is not individually experience rated, the individual patient is best off by using care as long as the value he places on the care exceeds the user cost he pays. Since all patients must pay collectively the full cost of care, all may be better off if they keep use below this level. But which of the two levels of output is the one the physician should choose in his role as agent? One of the advantages of the HMO may be precisely that it does cause the physician to behave *not* as the agent of his own patients, or of the fraction of the membership he treats, but rather as agent for the entire membership group.

Can this same kind of "group agency" be attained under fee-for-service? If the physician does completely control what happens to the patient, there is still some set of fees that can be found to induce him to supply exactly what he would supply if he were acting as agent for all patients. There is a stronger result, however. Given such a set of prices, the physician will provide this ideal amount of output to patients regardless of what individual patients do. Patients may want their physician to provide more output, but income-maximizing physicians will refuse to do so. Rather than levying user charges—copayments or deductibles —to discourage moral hazard, there is a scheme of reimbursement under fee-for-service that will have exactly the same effect as long as physicians are concerned, even if only slightly, about the aggregate well-being of their patients. If the fee structure is incentive neutral, physicians may even take differences in patient preferences into account to some extent, since doing so will improve patient well-being.

This abstract discussion can be illustrated with some examples. Consider those commonly cited examples of "overprovision" under fee-for-service: surgery and hospitalization in general. The physician's net income per hour worked is likely to be greater if he performs surgery than if he does not. It is therefore not surprising that there may be "excessive surgery" under fee-for-service, or that this rate can be reduced by capitation. What is not generally recognized, however, is that with a sufficiently low relative fee for surgery, this incentive could also be made to disappear. The emphasis here is on *relative* fees; an alternative to cutting fees for performing surgery would be to raise the fee for other procedures, such as consultation.

A second way of reducing marginal net real income (MNRI) is to raise opportunity costs; in addition to taxing the use of inputs, this could be done by increasing the number of hours worked per physician. Fewer surgeons should lead to incentives to perform less surgery, because the opportunity cost of each surgeon's time—the value of lost leisure—will be greater if he has less leisure. It is interesting to note that HMOs typically follow both of these strategies: they pay salaries or profit shares, which may imply zero or negative real net income from additional surgery, and they hire fewer surgeons relative to population served.

If a physician hospitalizes a patient for treatment of a given condition, he usually benefits in three ways: (1) he may be able to charge (and have insurance cover) a higher fee for procedures performed in hospital; (2) it may take less of his time to see patients in the hospital rather than in the office or at home, and yet his fee for a follow-up visit may be the same or greater; (3) as indicated in chapter 3, he may be able to substitute insured hospital inputs for uninsured inputs which he would provide. All of these reasons lead to a higher MNRI from hospitalization. The cure, again, is some reduction in MNRI—paying the same for a procedure regardless of where performed (or even possibly less if the procedure is performed in the hospital), paying less for visits which take less time, and perhaps some method of charging the physician for additional hospital inputs.[15] Where the user price of hospital treatment is below that of ambulatory treatment because the insurance only covers inpatient expenses, then the patient will still have an incentive to seek overprovision, even if physician incentives are rationalized. In such a case, as noted above, the notion of agency is ambiguous, and conflict between physician and patient may arise. Here moral hazard cannot be controlled directly. But at least for those outputs equally covered by insurance, restructuring of fees to yield, on average, approximately equal MNRI might go a long way toward reducing some of the abuses under fee-for-service.

Why Are Fees Out of Line?

In order for such a policy suggestion to succeed, one needs to have some idea of the forces which lead to the initial pattern of fees. Why *are* the MNRI per hour different for different outputs? One would have expected that the return to any input in different uses would tend to be equalized. Suppliers would devote time to the higher-yielding output, causing its price to fall and the price of other outputs to rise. Why hasn't this happened?

For those outputs whose physician fees are covered by insurance, it is easy to see why prices do not fall. Cutting price would not increase a surgeon's volume of business, even if he wanted to produce more output. This would still not prevent equalization if there were an unlimited amount of insured business. But there clearly is not enough surgery to permit all physicians who are licensed to perform it to do so.

Why do insurance plans not permit the fees they pay to fall? Perhaps it is because some physician insurances are provided by physician-dominated firms. To provide a complete explanation here would take us far from the main line of our argument. The only purpose here is to point out that insurance fee schedules may be the ultimate cause of over-provision of many physician services.

At a policy level, there are three broad strategies for remedying over-provision under fee-for-service. MNRI can be reduced either by cutting price or by raising unit cost. A cut in fees paid by third parties would accomplish the former, while a reduction in the number of physicians in specialties in which there is too much output would accomplish the latter. A third strategy involves making the demand for physician services used to produce insured outputs more elastic. Payment of indemnities, for example, makes price cutting pay, and so may lead to lower prices.

In summary, it is not fee-for-service as such that yields incentives for overprovision; rather, it is the level of existing fees for some procedures. Change the fees, either by lowering some or by raising others, and the overprovision will disappear. An additional corrective is that the total stock of physician input must be efficiently utilized; otherwise the specific examples of overuse we now see may be converted to a general problem of overuse of all physicians' services. Somewhat surprisingly, writers on the subject of incentives have generally ignored the flexibility available under a fee-for-service system. Monsma has given perhaps the most extensive treatment of the effect of what he calls "marginal revenue" on physician choice of output, but he has only a confused footnote exploring the possibility of how the MNRI under fee-for-service might be reduced.[16] He correctly says that, since marginal gross revenue is zero under capitation, MNRI there must be lower than under fees which yield positive MNRI. This yields the prediction that output should be less under capitation, but it does not answer the objection that output under capitation may be too low. In the absence of perfect competition, fee-for-service payment can still provide ideal incentives.

Changing the Fee Structure

There are two related objections to the notion that fee-for-service, with radically restructured fees, could be used to provide optimal incentives. It may be argued that the changes in fees may be so large as to (1) be infeasible or (2) if feasible, impractical because of the large reductions in some specialists' incomes they imply. For example, given the current level of MNRI for surgery, equalizing returns from surgery and consultation would probably imply enormous fees for consultation —perhaps $200 for a half-hour visit. Up to a point, this change might result not in less surgery, but just more consultation, if excess surgical capacity is sufficiently large. Conversely, cutting surgical fees to equalize MNRI might involve hefty cuts. Even if these were feasible, the consequent reduction in surgeons' incomes might, again up to a point, induce them to desire to do *more*, rather than less surgery than at present in order to keep their incomes up to their accustomed levels. A still further reduction in fees could reduce this incentive, but at the cost of a still less palatable reduction in income.

There are two kinds of responses to these objections. One is to note that they only represent the obvious consequences of erroneous manpower policy. Paying surgeons to do consultation may look expensive, but it may be less costly than having them use their time performing surgery, given that too many surgical specialists have been trained. The second is to note that in the long run, "appropriate" levels of physician-specialist incomes can be combined with "appropriate" incentives only if "appropriate" numbers of specialists are trained. In the interim, one might be able to obtain consent to a substantial reduction in fees by proposing to supplement fees with lump-sum payments to those physicians in specialties thought to be in excess supply. In order to get from a "wrong" fee-for-service system to a proper system, it may be necessary to use partial salary-capitation reimbursement for a time, but always as a supplement to a fee-for-service system.

5   The Availability Effect: Empirical Results

This chapter has two purposes: first, to compare the "information manipulation" version of the availability effect argument that was developed in chapter 4 with alternative explanations that have been or might be developed to explain the effect. The intent here is to develop suggestions for distinguishing empirically between the models, and to spell out the different implications of accepting any particular model. Second, this chapter will develop and use an empirical technique to test for the presence and causes of the availability effect.

Medical Need, Availability Effect, and the Economic Concept of Demand

The discussion of the availability effect in almost all of the noneconomic literature has implicitly been based on the principle of "medical need" or what Fuchs has called the "monotechnic" point of view.[1] In its strongest form this principle asserts that, for any set of preexisting symptoms or complaints, there is a unique, appropriate, and necessary course of treatment, which has unique resource or input requirements. Neither individual preferences nor costs are relevant. For example, there is a specific set of indications for appendectomy or hernia repair. If the indications are present, the procedure "ought" to be demanded and performed. If they are absent, it ought not to be performed. It follows that, for a population with a given distribution of symptoms, there should be a unique number of procedures which ought to be performed, and a unique set of inputs which ought to be used to perform those procedures. While adherents of this view recognize that there may sometimes be vagueness about the necessity of a particular procedure, they do not usually discuss what will or should then determine what is to be done, other than to suggest that additional clinical trials would settle the matter.[2]

The critical feature of the medical need approach is that what should be done is held to depend only upon the patient's physical and mental condition. It follows therefore that if the presence of inputs, of surgical specialists for example, is correlated with use when the prevalence of conditions is known or assumed to be constant, there is prima facie evidence of "demand" or use creation. If surgical rates vary when surgical manpower varies but surgically treatable pathology does not, excess resources must be creating "unnecessary" use. Note that this approach blends or combines normative and positive aspects: demand creation occurs when use varies for reasons for which it ought not.

The economic approaches to be discussed below differ from the medical need approach in that they permit use to be determined by more than just the patient's physical condition and possibly some socioeconomic characteristics. In particular, his tastes or desires, the price (real and monetary) that he pays, and the resources at his disposal are held to be things which affect his use. More than this, there is often the implicit normative judgment that, at least in principle and in some situations, these variables *ought* to affect what he gets. In this approach, then, demand creation requires one to look at *both* health or condition indicators and economic variables before attributing any residual influence to an availability effect.

Viewed as a positive theory of behavior, the economic approach is much less likely to label a given act of behavior as demand creation. Suppose, for instance, a patient has insurance which covers all hospital costs. Suppose there is some newly developed, exotic, and expensive procedure for which facilities have just been installed and which promises him a positive but slight improvement in his expected health. If the patient uses that procedure, this would not be regarded as demand creation; it should only be regarded as satisfaction of his (large) demand at a zero price; supply is responding to demand. The installation of the equipment does not create the demand for improvement in health; it is only the supply response to previously unsatisfied demand. A physician would not be acting in the role of agent for his patient if he did not recommend the procedure. The physician might, especially if he is somewhat unorthodox, recognize the true waste involved in this transaction, and so label it the "technological imperative," but it would not be a manifestation of demand creation. If the patient, supposing he were truly informed, chose *not* to have the procedure done, but the physician manipulated information to get the patient's approval, *that* would be regarded as demand creation.

Economic Theories of the Availability Effect

In what follows I will concentrate on availability effects for physicians' services. Hospital care will be considered in a later chapter. The data will not permit empirical analysis of other types of medical care.

There are four kinds of theoretical explanations of the availability effect to be investigated:

1. The availability effect arises from statistical properties of the estimation procedure.

2. The availability effect represents the response of use to changes in the time or convenience cost of care.

3. Medical services are subject to chronic excess demand, and care is rationed by physicians on the basis of the interest or severity of cases, but excess demand is reduced when the availability of physicians is increased.

4. Physicians create demand by manipulating the information they provide to consumers; when more physicians are present, they alter information to induce consumers to use more care.

These explanations are obviously not mutually exclusive. Consequently, a test which supports one theory does not necessarily disprove another. Moreover, because a number of natural theoretical variables will not be measured (and may not be measurable) directly, proxy variables will have to be selected. As a result, the failure of an empirical test to confirm a theory may only indicate that inappropriate proxy variables were chosen, not that the theory itself is incorrect.

Data Selection and Statistical Properties

It is clear that trying to estimate a separate availability effect from aggregate data will involve a severe identification problem. The demand equation of interest is of the general form

(1) $$Q_D = D(P, X, Z)$$

where Q_D is quantity of some medical input demanded, P is its (user) price, X is a vector of other demand parameters, and Z is a vector of measures of input availabilities. In most demand studies, observations on use per capita and availability have been taken from geographic aggregates.

The problem with such an approach is that not all of the right-hand side variables are exogenous, nor is (1) the sole equation determining observed use Q. One of the other equations would, for example, be a production function:

(2) $$Q = Q(Z)$$

If some demand variables are omitted, if supply responds to demand, and if more inputs are needed to supply this output, there will necessarily be more use where there are more inputs. But there is no independent causal effect. Input availability does not cause more use; rather, when people desire more use, more inputs become available.

It has been noted less frequently that ostensible demand creation could also arise because of measurement error in demand variables. Suppose, as is very common, user price is measured only imperfectly. But suppose that supply responds well to an increase in quantity demanded induced by a decline in user price. In effect, supply availability may be a better proxy measure of true user price than is measured price. In such a case, price elasticity would be underestimated (because of errors-in-variables bias) and the demand creation effect would be overestimated. These problems will tend to be most severe when observations consist of aggregates over the size of a market area (e.g., a state or SMSA).

In such cases there is likely to be still another source of bias if population is measured accurately, and data on use and input availability are taken from the same source. For instance, hospital admissions and hospital beds are usually drawn from the same American Hospital Association survey. But such surveys may omit some possible observations— e.g., the AHA survey omits both Veterans Administration hospital beds and admissions to such hospitals. Then the coefficient on the independent variable will again be biased upward as a measure of the effects of inputs on *total* use.

In general, if equation (1) were estimated using actual values of Z, it is clear that the coefficient on Z might be biased upward. This bias might be avoided by using predicted values of the Z variables in a two-stage procedure. But there may still be problems: there may not be an exogenous variable in the supply equation with which to identify the demand equation. To see this, consider the most fully specified model, that of Fuchs and Kramer.[3] In a technical sense, their approach is free of the omitted demand variable problem because they treat physicians per capita (MD^*) as an endogenous variable, and so estimate the demand equation in which MD^* enters by $2SLS$. They therefore use a predicted value for MD^* rather than the actual value, and this predicted value should be free from correlation with any omitted demand variables. However, the exogenous variables which are used in the first stage to predict MD^* are either explicitly demand variables, or, what is more serious, they are variables which might not really be exogenous, but rather would themselves be correlated with the omitted demand variables.

For example, one of the most important variables in the MD^* equation is hospital beds per capita. But as was argued above, and as will be developed in more detail in chapter 6, it seems more reasonable to suppose that beds and physician time are jointly demanded to produce hospital output. Neither physicians nor beds are exogenous. This effect is even stronger in the Fuchs-Kramer study, since interstate variation in their measure of physician visits per capita (the dependent variable in the demand equation) depends strongly on variation in hospital bed-days per capita, because physician hospital visits are estimated by using the number of bed-days. For both of these reasons, it is likely that much of the positive relationship between MD^* and beds arises from their mutual dependence on omitted demand variables. The other important predictor of MD^* is the number of medical schools in the state (*not* medical schools per capita, or per physician; apparently medical schools are a public good as far as physicians are concerned). It would again appear to be a reasonable conjecture that, if more medical schools in a state do mean more physicians, those states with unusually high demands for physicians' services would be expected to have more medical schools. Again, this variable could be correlated with omitted demand variables.

This is a specific illustration of the general difficulty of finding "truly exogenous" supply variables for a product whose output does not depend on weather or geography. A better choice would have been some determinants of real physician income, such as temperature, extent of urban amenities, or golf courses per capita, or possibly some measures of governmental restrictions on physician flow. Fuchs and Kramer did try some of these variables, but apparently they were not strongly related to MD. In a more recent study of the demand for surgical services, Fuchs was able to relate the surgeon stock to hotel expenditures per capita as a proxy for locational desirability.[4]

One way to mitigate these problems is to avoid aggregated data. That is, instead of using per capita demand in a market area, which is surely going to be related to area-wide levels of omitted variables, one could use as observations the quantities demanded by individuals. It is less likely that the number of physicians will respond appreciably to unusually high or low demands by a single individual. One can only say less likely, not unlikely, since it is possible that any omitted variables might affect all persons in an area in a similar way. If, for instance, all or almost all people in South Dakota have unusually low demands for physicians' services, perhaps because of a common ethnic background, then the omitted variable problem returns. If however, the variance within areas of some characteristic is sufficiently large, and especially if it is large relative to the variance across areas, input availability can safely be treated as exogenous to a given individual. For these reasons, and also because of other desirable aspects of the data, individual observations will be used in the empirical analysis which follows.

Nonmoney Price and the Availability Effect

There is one omitted demand variable which should be given special attention. Suppose the number of physicians in an area is increased exogenously. The money price of their services may fall. But, in addition, the time and inconvenience cost of seeing a physician is likely to be reduced. Distances will be shortened, the possibility of waiting in queues reduced, and so on. As Acton[5] has shown, the time cost of ambulatory physicians' services may be large relative to the money price or cost. Consequently, even with money price held constant, an alteration in input availability may have a substantial effect on use if it affects the time cost of care. (Quality might also be affected.)

It may be possible to construct a test to suggest whether the availability effect arises from a change in the time cost of care. Let the total price of a unit of care be given by

$$(3) \qquad P = P_M + Wt$$

where P_M is the (user) money price, t is the time spent per unit of care obtained, and W is a measure of the opportunity cost of time.

Suppose all buyers wait approximately the same length of time. Suppose that increases in physicians per capita reduce waiting time by the same amount for all persons. Newhouse and Phelps[6] have shown that

$$(4) \qquad \eta_{qt} = \frac{Wt}{P_M + Wt} \, \epsilon$$

where η_{qt} is the elasticity of demand with respect to time and ϵ is the elasticity of demand with respect to total (money plus time) price. It follows directly that changes in physician stock will reduce time cost by a larger amount for high wage persons. Since time cost is a larger fraction of total cost for high wage persons, equation (4) implies that, if ϵ is the same for all persons, the elasticity of use with respect to physician stock η_{qm} will vary positively with W. While it is likely that higher wage persons will seek medical care which has a higher money cost and a lower time cost, it seems reasonable to suppose that money cannot be substituted for time to such an extent that total time cost will be less. (If P_M equalled zero for a low-income person, then η_{qt} would equal ϵ, and would be greater than η_{qt} for other persons. However, persons in households with incomes low enough to make them eligible for Medicaid are omitted from the sample that will be used.)

Since in practice W and income often vary together, and ϵ may decline with income, availability elasticities may not differ significantly. In the empirical work, I shall make some attempt to control for income while W varies. Note finally that if, instead of being constant elasticity, the demand curve is assumed to be approximately linear in P and q, then ϵ will *increase* as W (and P) increase, making the predicted variation in η_{qm} with W even more likely.

Time cost may also be relevant for understanding differences in the availability effect between urban and rural areas. It is often alleged that there is a relative "shortage" of physicians in rural areas. Indeed, the per capita number of physicians is substantially less in such areas. Time cost may therefore be high in such areas. If time cost is higher in rural areas and if relative money prices are the same in rural and urban areas, a given percentage change in physician stock should produce a larger percentage change in total price in rural areas. To the extent that the availability effect operates through a change in time cost, the elasticity of use of care with respect to physician stock would therefore surely be positive and probably greater in rural than in urban areas. While nominal money prices are lower in rural areas, so is the cost of living, so that relative prices may be sufficiently uniform to permit this test.

Excess Demand

Excess demand exists when the quantity demanded of some service exceeds the quantity supplied at a given price. If excess demand for physicians' services exists at current prices, it is possible that an increase in supply of physicians may cause the observed quantity used to increase with no change in money prices. The case is clearest and neatest when excess demand occurs because of price controls imposed on exogenously determined input supplies. If price is below the market-clearing price, quantity supplied will fall short of quantity demanded. Now let there be an exogenous increase in inputs available to produce care (physicians, beds). The quantity used at the fixed price will increase: this might be called an availability effect.

Of course, if price controls exist everywhere (though at different prices below the equilibrium one), the "demand" elasticity that will be observed empirically will have the wrong sign, since the estimated relationship will actually represent points on a supply curve. If price controls exist in some places from which observations are taken but not others, one may observe *both* a negative demand elasticity and an "availability effect," neither of which will be accurately measured.

The price control model is not very realistic, since, except for the Economic Stabilization Program and some kinds of Blue Shield reimbursement mechanisms (now largely disused), prices are not fixed. One can argue that if prices respond slowly to excess supply or demand, the actual situation may approximate price controls. But this leaves the uncomfortable questions of why prices respond so slowly, and whether one observes equilibrium or disequilibrium in a cross section.[7]

A more complete answer is provided by arguing that there are *reasons* why the price might stay below the market-clearing level. All of these reasons involve entering either the magnitude of excess demand or the price itself in the provider's utility function. In what follows I will first consider alternative theories of physician behavior that might be constructed to explain the existence of permanent excess demand.

Feldstein[8] was the first economist to suggest that physicians may get utility from excess demand; this was one of his explanations for the upward slope of his estimated "demand" curve for physicians' services. (He also argued that lower prices give physicians utility.) The notion is that physicians maintain a queue in order to be able to select "interesting" or urgent cases.

Feldstein appealed to the existence of a chronic doctor shortage since 1946 as evidence for the existence of such utility functions. Exactly what the evidence is for this shortage, and its dimensions, was nowhere stated. However, it will still be useful to present a model of equilibrium nonprice rating.

I assume that each physician has a utility function of the form $U = U(Y, \alpha)$ where Y is money income and α is the fraction of total cases seen that is regarded as interesting. I assume that hours of work are fixed at L, and that output (number of cases seen) depends only on hours of work. Each physician is assumed to be confronted with a pro-rata share of the market demand curve. Of the total demand (or per physician demand) at each price, the fraction α_D of cases is interesting. However, the physician is assumed to be unable to charge different prices for interesting and uninteresting cases. For example, it may not be possible for the patient (or physician) to identify beforehand which initial visits will be for interesting conditions. Thus, if each physician sets price at the level which clears the market at $Q_D = Q_S = Q(L)$, then $\alpha = \alpha_D$. However, if physicians value interesting cases, they may be willing to reduce prices below the market clearing level. That is, the only way to induce demand for initial and subsequent visits for interesting cases may be to set an initial price below the market-clearing level, and then select interesting cases from the queue thus generated. The marginal equilibrium condition here (holding quantity supplied Q_S constant) is:

$$\frac{U_\alpha}{U_Y} \frac{\alpha_D \partial Q_D / \partial P}{Q_S} = Q_S$$

where U_α is the marginal utility of the proportion of interesting cases, and U_Y is the marginal utility of income. It is easiest to explain this condition by considering a small change in price. The benefit from reducing price by one dollar is a gain in the fraction of interesting cases of $\alpha_D \dfrac{\partial Q/\partial P}{Q_S}$. But the cost is a reduction in income of Q_S. The physician will create excess demand for his services as long as the benefit from doing so exceeds the cost.

Since the cost of cutting price by one dollar, or Q_S, is positive for even the initial price reduction from the market-clearing income-maximizing level, it is possible that a physician who values interesting cases may still decide *not* to cut the price. The cost may just be too high. But if he does decide to cut price, the effects of such behavior may be to increase his utility, and price may settle to some value below the market-clearing price. Now let the number of physicians be increased. If price is held constant and if α is held constant, income will decline. If α is a normal good, each physician will reduce his desired level of α by drawing down his queue. (The initial price is likely to no longer be the equilibrium price.) Total output will increase, but the *increase in output will consist entirely of uninteresting cases.* This discussion shows a way of determining whether any observed availability effect may be attributed to this cause. In particular, the elasticity of use with respect to the number of physicians per capita should be less for cases labeled as interesting, or for persons with such cases, than for uninteresting cases.

The "interest" or "severity" on the basis of which rationing occurs is, of course, that which is perceived by the physician. Insofar as there are a priori reasons why physicians and patients might differ in their estimates of severity for particular kinds of cases, then another test of this kind of theory would involve determining whether the response for those kinds of cases which physicians do not deem to be severe is larger than for those cases which physicians do regard as severe. Such a test would require proxying severity by symptoms or by diagnosis, or by physician and patient attitudes toward symptoms and diagnosis.

Alternative bases for rationing other than severity yield alternative predictions about differences in the availability effect. It is possible, for example (as also suggested by Feldstein), that excess demand may arise if price enters the physician's utility function. Suppose demand increases for a type of care for which a critical physician input is in perfectly inelastic supply. A price rise could reequate demand and supply, but physicians may recognize that its only function is to transfer income from patients to physicians. Accordingly, they may neglect to raise prices, and ration on the basis of severity or interest. But the higher patients' incomes are relative to physicians' incomes, the less this kind of benevolent rationing is likely to occur. Thus one would predict that the response of use to availability should differ by severity, but that these differences should be greater the lower the relative incomes of patients. If severity itself enters the physician's utility function, there would be no such difference.

The precise determination of whether excess demand exists or not is difficult because queues do not necessarily mean that price is too low, any more than the existence of inventories means that the price is too high. When demand is stochastic, a profit-maximizing firm may choose to hold inventories, or to permit queues to develop; either way the production process is smoothed out. Which strategy is chosen depends, roughly speaking, on which is cheaper. Having groceries wait for people in the supermarket rather than vice versa makes sense if the costs of maintaining inventories are less than the costs of delay. Having people wait for doctors rather than vice versa makes sense if the cost of doctors' time exceeds that of the cost of patients' waiting time. What is actually chosen is some mix of queues and inventories: there are occasional delays at the supermarket, and doctors sometimes have time for a cup of coffee. *If* prices could be adjusted with this variation in demand, some (but probably not all) queues would disappear; but such adjustment is probably itself too costly. One can be certain that excess demand exists only if there is *always* a queue, and it is not clear that this obtains even for "busy" doctors.

One final question is whether the behavior predicted by these theories might also be predicted by, or at least consistent with, long-run profit-maximizing behavior on the parts of physicians. Unfortunately for the purposes of hypothesis testing, the answer seems to be yes.

It may be, for instance, that most people have a kind of implicit contract with their physician. Because it is too costly to vary prices with urgency and demand, the physician agrees to let the patient jump the queue at no increase in price for serious illness if the patient will wait (patiently?) in the queue when the complaint is nonurgent. This permits the physician to even out his patient flow, thus increasing his productivity and lowering the price he needs to charge. Thus it is possible to concoct a profit-maximizing explanation of both (1) the regular doctor and (2) taking the most serious cases first. Hospitals will do the same if they do what physicians want.

Measuring Information Manipulation

In the information manipulation theory, the demand equation of interest has the general form

$$Q^{ij}{}_D = Q(\tilde{P}^{ij}, X^i, A^j)$$

where $Q^{ij}{}_D$ is the quantity of a given medical service demanded by person i in area j, $\tilde{P}^{ij}$ is the user price (net of insurance) paid by person i, X^i is a vector of person i's demand characteristics (including his state of health, and A^j is the level of accuracy he experiences. It is assumed that A^j is the same for all persons in a given area.

It will be possible to obtain reasonable approximations of Q_D, $\tilde{P}$, and X. But A cannot be measured directly. Instead, as suggested by the earlier discussion, the level of accuracy chosen by the representative physician will depend upon the gross price level, the quantity that each physician can sell at that price, and the level of the physician's subjective marginal opportunity cost. I will assume that the marginal cost curve is the same for all providers. With gross price P^j held constant, total quantity demanded in an area depends on the mean area-wide values $\bar{X}^j$ of the demand parameters (including others' insurance coverage). The demand per physician then depends on the number of physicians. Thus we can write:

(2) $$A^j = A(P^j, MD^{*j}, \bar{X}^j)$$

where MD^{*j} is the stock of physicians per capita in area j and P^j is the gross price received by physicians in area j. Note that A is greater the larger the demand per physician. So while an individual's demand for physicians' services would be greater the sicker he is, it would be smaller the sicker everyone else in his community is, because in the latter case the physician would have less incentive to create demand.

Substituting the equation for A into the demand function gives

(3) $$Q_D{}^{ij} = Q(\tilde{P}^{ij}, X^i, \bar{X}^j, MD^{*j}, P^j)$$

Since $\tilde{P}^{ij} = INS^i P^j$, where INS^i is the fraction of i's expenditure not covered by insurance, the actual estimating equation will be

(3') $$Q^{ij}{}_D = Q(INS^i, P^j, X^i, \bar{X}^j, MD^{*j})$$

Since P^j has effects on consumer demand both directly through the user price and indirectly through incentives for demand creation, it is not desirable to impose the constraint that changes in INS^i and P^j which have the same influence on $\tilde{P}^{ij}$ should have the same influence on demand. In particular, changing $\tilde{P}^{ij}$ by changing INS^i should have a larger effect on quantity demanded than that from changing P^j, since changes in the prices paid to physicians provide offsetting incentives to create additional demand. In the data to be used there is no measure of the marginal or average fraction of expense covered by insurance, only an indication of whether or not the individual is covered by hospital and/or medical-surgical insurance. A dummy variable for INS is therefore used in the regressions. This procedure is equivalent to assuming that all persons who have insurance have the same coverage.

Target Income

A final kind of theory that contains elements of all of the preceding ones is the so-called "target income" theory. This theory was first suggested by Newhouse and Sloan,[9] but has received its most extensive development by Evans.[10] In its simplest and most naive form, the theory assumes that physicians have target money incomes and target workloads they wish to achieve. Both are chosen with reference to what is acceptable or usual in the community and in the profession. Productivity and the level of other inputs held constant, the target workload determines output Q. Given input prices and Q, the physician then chooses the gross output price that achieves the target income. If the Q chosen in this way exactly equals the Q corresponding to this gross price on some market demand curve, then demand is just satisfied. If Q is less than the quantity demanded, excess demand prevails. If Q is greater than the quantity demanded, actual Q will be increased as physicians "order extra work for patients, perform unnecessary or marginally necessary operations, or recall patients for extra visits."[11] Increases in the number of physicians will in either case result in an increase in actual Q at any price—an availability effect will be observed.

In its simplest version, the target income theory is consistent with an availability effect which arises *either* from the drawing down of excess demand or from demand creation. It simply makes observed demand depend on the number of physicians. If a distinction is to be made between a target income theory and any other theory, that distinction must be based on a presumed fixity in the incomes, real or money, that physicians desire.

If desired or target income is assumed to be fixed, the theory makes a definite qualitative empirical prediction which permits it to be distinguished from maximizing models. It predicts that an exogenous increase in gross price will lead to a *reduction* in the quantity of services per capita supplied and used. For if quantity were held constant, then income would rise. To keep it at the target level, quantity must fall.[12] The information-manipulation theory, however, is consistent with the finding of a positive or zero effect if the substitution effect of a price increase (which represents a greater reward for more business) offsets the income effect.

While Evans seemed initially to support the naive target income theory,[13] his "more extended model" allowed actual workload to depart from desired workload. More importantly, he allowed desired workloads to be a positive function of price, which makes it possible for price and quantity used to be positively related. He used casual empiricism on the Canadian experience to suggest that the relationship will still usually be negative, but the "extended" theory as such cannot be refuted. Indeed, as Sloan and Feldman have shown,[14] *any* outcome with respect to the relationship between physician stock and price or aggregate use would be possible under the "extended" theory.

These alterations make Evans' models indistinguishable from the demand creation model discussed in chapter 4; they rob the target income approach of any distinctive qualitative empirical predictions. In order to preserve this distinction, in what follows I shall regard the target income approach as the initial, naive model. Evans' "more extended model" will instead be identified with the information manipulation theory.

Data Sources and Variable Measurement

In this section some empirical tests of alternate theories of the availability effect will be provided. The basic source of data on individual use and individual characteristics is the 1970 Health Interview Survey of the National Center for Health Statistics.[15] This survey consists of the results of a questionnaire administered to about 110,000 persons in 39,000 families on their health, use of medical care during the past year, and socioeconomic characteristics, including insurance coverage. From A.M.A. and A.H.A. data sources, I obtained information on the number of physicians of various types, hospital beds, and gross prices of hospital and physician services in the "primary sampling units" (PSUs) from which the sample was drawn. PSUs are counties, groups of counties, or SMSAs. For 22 large SMSAs that are identified on the tape, the actual values of the PSU-level variables could be used. For the other PSUs the National Center for Health Statistics attached a set of decile rank orders of each of the variables to each of the PSU codes. I then substituted for the decile rank orders the population-weighted mean values of each of the variables for each combination of decile rank orders. In most cases, this procedure will associate a unique set of values for the area variables with each PSU. The variables used in the empirical work are as follows:

Dependent Variables

Three measures of utilization:

1. Physician visits, last 12 months. This includes telephone calls but excludes visits to hospital inpatients. Because of the recall period, there may be some error in measurement.

2. Hospital episodes, last 12 months, in nonfederal, short term hospitals.

3. Average stay per episode (equals hospital days divided by hospital episodes).

Independent Variables and Abbreviations

Personal Variables:

1. Restricted activity days, last two weeks (RAD).

2. Number of chronic conditions (CONDS).
3. Age (AGE).
4. Sex, 1 if female (SEX).
5. Female of childbearing age dummy (F15–44).
6. Family size (FAMSZ).
7. Work status: whether individual is currently employed or not (WORKING).
8. No insurance coverage (NOINS): indicates whether the individual is covered by hospitalization or surgical insurance or Medicare or not. About half of the surveyed families were asked this question, so in most of the analysis only observations on persons who were asked this question were used. However, restricting the data set to families who answered the question would lead to small cell size for the high education group in all but the large metropolitan areas. Accordingly, an insurance coverage variable is not included for high education families in other metropolitan or rural areas.
9. Family income in 100's (FAMINC).

PSU Variables:

10. Office based M.D.'s per 100 persons (OBMD*).
11. Surgical specialists as a fraction of office-based M.D.'s (SURG/ MD).
12. General practitioners as a fraction of office-based M.D.'s (GP/ MD). The variables GP/OBMD and SURG/OBMD measure the proportion of total office-based physicians who are general practitioners and surgeons respectively. They capture any differences in the quality or characteristics of a typical patient visit, as well as differential specialty effects, if any, on demand creation.
13. Hospital based M.D.'s per 100 persons (HBMD*)—mainly residents, interns, and other hospital-salaried physicians.
14. Nonfederal short-term hospital beds per 100 persons (BEDS*).
15. Hospital cost per patient-day for nonfederal short-term hospitals in the PSU (HOSCOST).
16. Population density (POPDENS).
17. Physician office visit fee (MDFEE). Two measures are used. The fee measure used for all areas is the fee screen for Medicare patients for followup office visits. This screen is supposed to represent the seventy-fifth percentile of the prevailing distribution of fees in various geographic areas. However, since different procedures are used by different carriers to set up the fee screen, the accuracy of this measure is unknown. When there were different fees for general practitioners and specialists, a weighted average was used. For the 100 largest SMSAs, Mathematica, Inc. conducted a telephone survey in 1973 to ascertain

the fee for a routine office visit to a primary care practitioner,[16] and this measure should be an accurate index of fee levels for such services. Accordingly, results for office visits for the 22 largest cities are presented using the Mathematica prices as well as using the Medicare fee screens.

In principle, cost-of-living differences should be taken into account in estimating monetary variables (income and fees). A complete set of such indexes is available from the Bureau of Labor Statistics only for the large-city subsample, not for all other cities or for rural areas. A comparison of regressions using undeflated and deflated data for the large city subsample will suggest whether the absence of deflation biases coefficients on the variables of interest.

Classification of Results for Physician Visits

Results for physician visits are presented for several different data sets. First, persons are classified by the number of physicians in the market area in which they live: the 22 largest SMSAs, in which it would probably be very difficult for consumers to get reliable information on any individual physician; nonmetropolitan areas, in which such information is presumably easier to obtain; and other, smaller metropolitan areas, which might be expected to be intermediate.

The information manipulation theory would suggest that availability might have a greater influence in those large metropolitan areas in which individuals have difficulty determining the quality or accuracy of the advice which any individual physician provides. An excess demand theory, on the other hand, would predict that availability effects would be most likely to be observed in rural areas, where physician stock is lowest and excess demand presumably the greatest.

Second, results are presented for persons in households in which the heads have different levels of education. Education level is intended to be a proxy for the prior stock of information. In most of the analysis, results will be presented for two extremes of the distribution of educational attainment—persons in households in which heads are not high school graduates (low head education) and persons in households with heads with college degrees or better (high head education)—for the reasons discussed in chapter 4.

Where an availability effect is detected, the sample is further subdivided in ways which, it is hoped, correspond to differences suggested by other theories of the availability effect. The survey did not ask about wage income or hours, but it did ask whether or not the person was employed. It would seem reasonable to suppose that, money income held constant, adults who are working have a higher time cost than adults who are not. Another method of division is by number of chronic conditions, which may serve as proxy for illness severity or physician interest in the case.

Two alternative methods of estimation were used. Since there is a concentration of observations at zero, especially for the low education group, ordinary least squares regression on all observations would yield incorrect estimates. Tobit regression is usually the appropriate technique to be used.[17] However, there are reasons to fear that tobit may not be theoretically appropriate for the question being investigated here, as has been suggested by Newhouse and Phelps.[18] Physician advice can only influence use if the consumer first contacts the physician to seek his advice. The initial decision to seek advice should not be influenced by physician information; although physician availability may influence this decision, it will do so through changes in nonmoney price. Once a person has made at least one visit, then he will potentially have received some physician advice and be subject to an information effect. Accordingly, analysis of the subsample of persons with positive doctor visits is more likely to display an information effect than is analysis of the total sample. Of course, not all of the persons with positive numbers of visits will have been subject to information manipulation; there may be several initial visits, for a series of illnesses, included in the data. Moreover, the censoring issue discussed earlier suggests that those with positive visits may be more susceptible to information manipulation than those with no visits. Nevertheless, the set of those with positive visits may still be more appropriate for investigation of an availability effect than the full sample. Such analysis of nonzero observation can be done using OLS, since there is less of a concentration of observations at a lower limit.

Two kinds of person are omitted from the sample. Persons with household incomes below a poverty line are dropped because their use is likely to be covered by Medicaid and so not responsive to changes in fees. Those with more than 52 physician visits in a year are also dropped in order to avoid bias from extreme values.

The full specification described in the section "Measuring Information Manipulation" indicates that area demand variables as well as individual demand characteristics should be included in the equations. Several such area demand variables—percentage of population covered by Medicare, percentage of under-65 population with private health insurance (for the state in which the SMSA is located) and percentage of population under age 5—are available for the 22 large cities. Accordingly, results with regressions which include these variables are also presented.

Empirical Results: Physician Ambulatory Visits

The primary prediction of the information-manipulation theory is that alterations in accuracy should have less effect on those with sufficiently larger prior stocks of information. There are two primary proxies for incentives for alterations in accuracy suggested by the theory: the number of physicians per capita, and the gross price of a unit of output.

The two major questions of interest are: (1) whether availability effects are shown and (2) if effects are shown, whether they differ across educational groups. Table 5.1 shows the coefficients for OLS regressions of physician visits during the preceding 12 months for persons with positive physician visits. Different regressions are presented for persons in the two separate education groups and in three different geographic areas; means and standard deviations are shown in appendix table 1. Table 5.2 presents similar tobit regressions on the full sample of persons. For the reasons discussed above, the availability effect is most likely to be observed in the positive visits sample, and so these results will be discussed first.

Availability variables

The three availability variables are OBMD*, HBMD* and BEDS*. OBMD* has a significant and positive coefficient for the low education group in two out of three geographic areas. The size of the coefficient (and the elasticity) is much larger in the large urban areas than in the rural areas. For high education families, however, the coefficient on OBMD* is *negative* and significant for the large urban areas, and insignificant elsewhere. HBMD* tends to have the same sign as OBMD*, but to have a lower significance level. BEDS* is not usually significant. Application of an F-test for differences in the sets of coefficients across education groups finds that the set of coefficients on the two education groups is significantly different in all three area subsamples. In addition, the coefficients on OBMD* and HBMD* do differ significantly between the low and high education regressions in two of the three areas.

The remainder of the area variables are occasionally significant, but there is no consistent pattern. The proportion of physicians who are G.P.'s does not affect the ambulatory visit rate, while the proportion who are surgical specialists tends to depress the rate, but to a significant extent only for high education families. While none of the coefficients differs significantly across education groups, there is some weak evidence that surgeons may substitute away from ambulatory care toward hospital care. However, the results for the effect of surgeons on hospital use, to be presented later, do not confirm this suggestion. Another plausible explanation is that surgical specialists treat conditions with fewer ambulatory visits even when they do not substitute inpatient hospital stays. The physician's fee is not significant for high education families, but does have a significant and positive effect for the low education families in smaller metropolitan areas.

Other demand variables have generally expected coefficients. Both restricted activity days and number of chronic conditions are strongly related to the doctor visit rate. Older persons tend to make more visits as do females in general (in low education families) and females of childbearing age. Family size has a slight tendency to reduce the visit rate, while workers make fewer visits than nonworkers.

These results are consistent with the information manipulation theory of the availability effect. When an availability effect is observed, it is positive and significant for the low education families in two out of three areas. (The negative and significant effect of OBMD* for high education families in large cities may reflect a change in the quality or character of ' a visit when physicians are more plentiful.) There is also a *positive* and significant effect of price on use for low education families in the other

Table 5.1   **Physician Visits Regressions: Persons with Some Physician Visits**
(ordinary least squares)

| | Regression Coefficients (*t* statistics in parentheses) | | | | | |
| Independent Variable or Statistic | 22 Largest SMSAs | | Other SMSAs | | Nonmetropolitan Areas | |
	Low Head Education	High Head Education	Low Head Education	High Head Education	Low Head Education	High Head Education
RAD	.176	.280	.067	.212	.263	.370
	(4.15)	(4.69)	(1.59)	(3.90)	(6.93)	(6.54)
CONDS	2.21	1.81	1.60	1.63	1.60	1.50
	(17.4)	(12.3)	(13.8)	(13.8)	(15.7)	(12.83)
AGE LT 15	−.304	−.429	−.140	1.18	−.376	.304
	(−0.73)	(−0.97)	(−0.35)	(3.45)	(−1.07)	(0.83)
AGE 45–64	.986	.061	1.00	.172	1.06	.254
	(2.55)	(0.14)	(2.72)	(0.42)	(3.19)	(0.70)
AGE 65+	2.45	1.78	.722	1.83	.901	1.00
	(5.01)	(2.68)	(1.53)	(3.65)	(2.09)	(1.88)
SEX	.599	.229	.510	−.101	.451	−.455
	(2.16)	(0.70)	(1.93)	(−0.40)	(1.91)	(−1.74)
F 15–44	.636	.919	.849	1.51	1.20	1.38
	(1.39)	(1.90)	(1.97)	(4.02)	(3.10)	(3.48)
FAMSZ	−.066	−.064	−.052	−.190	−.071	−.230
	(−0.97)	(−0.88)	(−0.89)	(−3.39)	(−1.23)	(−3.66)
WORKING	−.712	−1.33	−.965	−.095	−.620	−1.05
	(−2.54)	(−4.14)	(−3.67)	(−0.60)	(−2.63)	(−3.89)
NOINS	.027	−.994	−.350	——	.517	——
	(0.08)	(−2.02)	(−1.26)	——	(2.19)	——
FAMINC	.001	−.004	.002	−.0001	.0003	−.001
	(0.30)	(−2.55)	(0.95)	(−0.03)	(0.27)	(−0.76)
GP/MD	3.03	−7.14	2.40	−.281	1.54	−1.89
	(0.56)	(−1.60)	(1.09)	(−0.12)	(1.37)	(−1.63)
SURG/MD	−7.00	−16.6	−5.89	−1.21	−.551	−4.63
	(−0.64)	(−1.66)	(−1.35)	(−0.28)	(−0.28)	(−2.09)
POPDENS	.019	.007	−.029	−.052	.173	−.053
	(1.09)	(0.38)	(−0.95)	(−2.12)	(2.62)	(−0.76)
MDFEE	−.125	.126	.178	.009	−.043	.010
	(−0.80)	(0.73)	(2.59)	(0.15)	(−0.28)	(1.14)

Table 5.1—*continued*

Independent Variable or Statistic	22 Largest SMSAs		Other SMSAs		Nonmetropolitan Areas	
	Low Head Education	High Head Education	Low Head Education	High Head Education	Low Head Education	High Head Education
HOSCOST	−.025	.019	−.019	−.003	.025	.045
	(1.79)	(1.28)	(−1.74)	(−0.42)	(2.56)	(0.78)
BEDS*	−2.29	−.370	−1.13	−2.13	−.968	.611
	(−0.87)	(−0.15)	(−0.95)	(−2.12)	(2.62)	(1.04)
HBMD*	14.0	−18.3	4.89	−.945	3.59	−7.93
	(1.59)	(−1.93)	(0.88)	(−.197)	(1.16)	(−2.88)
OBMD*	32.0	−25.8	−.902	3.55	5.79	.771
	(3.02)	(−2.44)	(−.134)	(0.56)	(2.53)	(0.62)
Constant	4.38	12.18	4.96	4.59	.523	5.31
	(0.65)	(2.22)	(1.73)	(1.78)	(0.13)	(3.92)
$\bar{R}^2$	.169	.140	.123	.101	.173	.131
n	3461	2189	2545	3184	3128	2562

Regression Coefficients (*t* statistics in parentheses)

F statistic for hypothesis of inequality of regression coefficients. ($F_{.01}$ [19, large n] = 1.88.)

2.38	2.46	2.85

NOTE: Means and standard deviations are shown in appendix table 2.

Table 5.2   **Physician Visits Regressions: All Persons (Tobit Regressions)**

Independent Variable or Statistic	22 Largest SMSAs		Other SMSAs		Nonmetropolitan Areas	
	Low Head Education	High Head Education	Low Head Education	High Head Education	Low Head Education	High Head Education
	Regression Coefficients (*t* statistics in parentheses)					
RAD	.506	.488	.349	.404	.566	.566
	(8.51)	(6.45)	(7.49)	(4.15)	(9.02)	(7.27)
CONDS	4.05	3.32	2.82	2.76	3.44	2.81
	(21.6)	(15.4)	(19.5)	(13.4)	(19.0)	(15.5)
AGE LT 15	1.59	1.37	.082	1.76	.954	1.69
	(2.90)	(2.50)	(0.19)	(3.06)	(1.73)	(3.48)
AGE 45–64	0.55	0.66	.091	.015	.129	.263
	(1.10)	(1.26)	(0.23)	(0.03)	(0.25)	(0.55)
AGE 65+	1.72	.825	−.464	1.16	−.072	.052
	(2.70)	(1.00)	(−0.92)	(1.39)	(−0.11)	(0.07)
SEX	.748	.093	1.12	.197	.770	−.777
	(2.05)	(0.23)	(3.94)	(0.46)	(2.07)	(−2.21)
F 15–44	2.05	2.70	.395	1.93	2.67	2.60
	(3.43)	(4.47)	(0.85)	(3.05)	(4.39)	(4.88)

Table 5.2—*continued*

Independent Variable or Statistic	22 Largest SMSAs		Other SMSAs		Nonmetropolitan Areas	
	Low Head Education	High Head Education	Low Head Education	High Head Education	Low Head Education	High Head Education
	Regression Coefficients (*t* statistics in parentheses)					
FAMSZ	−.332	−.262	−.209	−.261	−.257	−.331
	(−3.62)	(−2.74)	(−2.84)	(−2.76)	(−2.89)	(−3.76)
WORKING	−.173	−1.58	−.811	−.213	−.304	−1.04
	(−0.47)	(−3.83)	(−2.83)	(−0.49)	(−0.81)	(−2.85)
NOINS	−.219	−1.76	−.121	——	−1.59	.549
	(−0.55)	(−3.19)	(−0.39)	——	(−4.31)	(2.05)
FAMINC	.011	.000	.009	.003	.002	−.002
	(3.44)	(0.04)	(3.71)	(1.15)	(0.50)	(−0.98)
GP/MD	.800	−7.78	1.60	−2.89	−1.09	−.481
	(0.12)	(−1.40)	(0.66)	(−0.80)	(−0.60)	(−0.30)
SURG/MD	−6.09	−8.81	−3.60	−3.51	−5.71	−.612
	(−0.43)	(−0.71)	(−0.75)	(−0.49)	(−1.85)	(−0.20)
POPDENS	.042	.023	.011	−.067	−.008	−.119
	(1.83)	(0.87)	(0.35)	(−1.70)	(−0.94)	(−1.69)
MDFEE	−.363	−.327	.047	−.116	−.004	.143
	(−1.80)	(−1.51)	(0.53)	(−1.16)	(−0.31)	(1.95)
HOSCOST	−.066	.018	−.010	.016	.005	.006
	(−3.57)	(0.97)	(−0.93)	(1.08)	(2.82)	(0.51)
BEDS*	−8.87	−5.98	−.059	−1.34	−.525	.705
	(2.63)	(−2.07)	(−0.05)	(0.78)	(−0.45)	(0.90)
HBMD*	30.7	10.15	2.40	2.73	−3.20	−9.04
	(2.62)	(0.85)	(0.39)	(0.14)	(−0.65)	(−2.38)
OBMD*	45.7	−3.79	6.78	−.023	2.21	−.754
	(3.31)	(0.28)	(0.95)	(−0.00)	(0.26)	(−0.46)
Constant	6.06	8.15	−.225	2.81	−2.56	1.49
	(0.70)	(1.18)	(−0.07)	(0.67)	(−1.14)	(0.50)
Significance of chi-square statistic	.000	.000	.000	.000	.000	.000
n	5005	2693	3864	3950	4927	3323

NOTE: Means and standard deviations are shown in appendix table 1.

metropolitan areas, again offering evidence for demand creation (but against the naive target income theory).[19]

It is also worth noting that, although there is an availability effect for low education families in rural areas, that effect is much smaller than in large urban areas. Since rural areas are supposed to be areas of greatest physician "shortage," one could conclude either that the shortage is relatively mild, or that the potential for demand manipulation in such areas is limited by better consumer information on the accuracy of information provided by individual physicians.

The results of tobit analysis are shown in table 5.2. While these results are not conclusive, and while there is no precise way to test the hypothesis, the results are consistent with the notion that the effect of physician availability on whether or not people ever see a physician in a year can be different from the effect on the number of visits they make, given that they make at least one visit. While many of the coefficients are similar in sign, the tobit analysis does yield results for the high education/large urban group which are quite different from those for the persons in the same group with positive doctor visits. The insignificant coefficient of OBMD* in the tobit regressions may be a composite of a significant negative coefficient for those with positive visits and a positive effect on the probability of seeing a physician at all. (It might be possible to develop a statistical test, analogous to an F-test, to determine whether the structures of the OLS and tobit samples are different.) The availability variables in the other regressions tend to have similar signs in OLS and tobit specifications, as do the personal characteristic variables.

Because a large availability effect was detected for the large urban subsample, additional analysis was performed on it. First, variables measured in money were deflated by a cost-of-living index, with little change in results (table 5.3). Absence of such deflators for the other two area subsamples is therefore unlikely to affect results. Next, area-wide demand variables were added to the regressions. The variables added were (1) income per capita, (2) percentage of population over

Table 5.3	Physician Visit Regressions Using Deflated Money Variables, Area Demand Variables, and Alternative Price Measures: 22 Largest SMSAs, Persons with Some Visits					
Independent Variable or Statistic	Money Variables Deflated by Cost-of-living Index		Money Variables Deflated and Area Demand Variables Added		Mathematica Fee Estimates Used	
	Low Head Education	High Head Education	Low Head Education	High Head Education	Low Head Education	High Head Education
	Regression Coefficients (*t* statistics in parentheses)					
RAD	.257	.407	.253	.412	.256	.407
	(6.32)	(7.21)	(6.13)	(7.20)	(6.29)	(7.20)
CONDS	2.36	2.15	2.39	2.18	2.36	2.15
	(17.7)	(13.1)	(17.6)	(13.1)	(17.7)	(13.1)
AGE LT 15	−.159	−.163	−.343	−.069	−.163	−.174
	(−0.39)	(−0.37)	(−0.82)	(−0.16)	(−0.40)	(−0.40)
AGE 45–64	.807	−.007	.787	.065	.816	−.011
	(2.09)	(−0.02)	(2.01)	(0.15)	(2.11)	(−0.02)
AGE 65+	2.11	1.41	2.05	1.53	2.12	1.39
	(4.33)	(2.14)	(4.13)	(2.26)	(4.35)	(2.11)

Table 5.3—*continued*

Independent Variable or Statistic	Money Variables Deflated by Cost-of-living Index		Money Variables Deflated and Area Demand Variables Added		Mathematica Fee Estimates Used	
	Low Head Education	High Head Education	Low Head Education	High Head Education	Low Head Education	High Head Education
	Regression Coefficients (*t* statistics in parentheses)					
SEX	.593	.259	.659	.272	.592	:263
	(2.15)	(0.80)	(2.35)	(0.82)	(2.14)	(0.80)
F 15–44	.671	.889	.607	.873	.672	.880
	(1.46)	(1.84)	(1.32)	(1.78)	(1.47)	(1.82)
FAMSZ	−.100	−.090	−.080	−.079	−.098	−.087
	(−1.14)	(−1.17)	(−1.11)	(−1.00)	(−1.37)	(−1.13)
WORKING	−.848	−1.30	−.964	−1.17	−.857	−1.30
	(−3.02)	(−3.43)	(−3.39)	(−3.49)	(−3.06)	(−3.98)
NOINS	.028	−1.05	.037	−1.04	.014	−1.03
	(0.09)	(−2.32)	(0.12)	(−2.23)	(0.05)	(−2.29)
FAMINC	.002	−.004	.001	−.005	.002	−.004
	(0.70)	(−2.17)	(0.49)	(−2.37)	(0.20)	(−2.21)
GP/MD	7.30	−8.99	7.89	−14.3	5.98	−8.30
	(1.63)	(−2.16)	(1.43)	(−2.74)	(1.38)	(−1.95)
SURG/MD	3.20	−19.6	−1.22	−33.4	−1.87	−17.8
	(0.34)	(−0.78)	(−0.08)	(−2.36)	(−0.18)	(−1.79)
POPDENS	.009	−.006	.054	−.063	−.002	−.002
	(0.50)	(−0.31)	(1.61)	(−1.60)	(−0.10)	(−0.10)
MDFEE	−.040	.171	−.118	.445	.154	.103
	(−0.20)	(0.78)	(−0.49)	(1.65)	(0.54)	(0.34)
HOSCOST	−.024	.028	−.056	.034	−.030	.019
	(−1.46)	(1.49)	(−2.24)	(1.40)	(−1.83)	(1.20)
BEDS*	−1.60	.638	−1.69	1.79	−.215	−.241
	(−0.56)	(0.24)	(−0.43)	(0.50)	(−0.06)	(−0.08)
HBMD*	10.9	−14.9	8.80	−18.2	16.7	−15.4
	(1.23)	(−1.65)	(0.80)	(−1.56)	(1.65)	(−1.46)
OBMD*	34.6	−26.0	28.6	−29.2	30.5	−25.5
	(3.18)	(−2.13)	(2.08)	(−2.23)	(2.51)	(−1.96)
Inc. Per Cap.			−.001	−.001		
			(−1.02)	(−0.84)		
% over 65			−.163	−.256		
			(−0.75)	(−1.07)		
% with insurance (in state)			−.067	.044		
			(−1.69)	(1.03)		
Constant	−1.00	11.1	14.4	16.6	−.334	11.8
	(−0.17)	(2.13)	(1.06)	(1.23)	(−0.17)	(2.13)
$\bar{R}^2$	.173	.146	.177	.147	.173	.146
n*	3461	2189	3311	2126	3461	2189

*Because of the absence of data for some areas in which the SMSA crosses state boundaries, the sample size is slightly reduced for the regressions with area demand variables.

65, and (3) percentage of population with some health insurance. As shown in table 5.3, this addition decreased the estimated magnitude of the availability effect, but the changes were small. Coefficients on all of the areawide variables were negative, as expected, although the only significant coefficient was for areawide family income in the high education subsample. It does not appear that omission of such variables makes a substantial difference, and an F-test indicates that the set of area demand variables does not significantly increase the explanatory power of the regression. Finally, use of the possibly more accurate prices from the Mathematica survey yielded approximately the same coefficients as the use of the other price measure.

Because of the large positive availability effect for the low education/ large urban subsample, that subsample was further disaggregated to examine alternative theories of the availability effect. The information-manipulation theory is not refuted by the chronic/nonchronic illness distinction. As shown in table 5.4, the increase in use in response to more physicians is obviously not confined to, nor is it larger for, those with zero chronic conditions. Of course, we cannot be sure that those with chronic conditions are really more severely ill, or that their visits are more desired by physicians, although Friedman offers evidence to suggest that they are.[20] It is also possible, as suggested by Grossman and Rand, that time costs are greater for the chronically ill because they are more severely disabled.[21]

The comparison between the effect on working and nonworking adults fails to support the time cost theory (table 5.4). The coefficients and elasticities on OBMD* are not statistically different between those who work and those who do not. There is no evidence that the response of working adults to a reduction in the availability of physicians (as a proxy for time cost) is greater than that of nonworking adults.

Is the Availability Effect Important for Ambulatory Care?

Determining the reason for any observed availability effect was the primary purpose of this study. However, the results appear to be consistent not only with the hypothesis that the response of use to physician availability differs across education groups, but even with the hypothesis that the effect is important only for low education families.

In order to get an idea of the overall importance of the availability effect for ambulatory care, persons with other levels of education were added to the sample and the regressions rerun. In principle, it would have been preferable to permit interactions between education or location and all of the independent variables, but the large sample size made

Table 5.4   **Physician Visits Regressions, Persons with Some Visits in Households with Low Head Education: 22 Largest SMSAs, Selected Subsamples**

| Statistic Independent Variable or | Regression Coefficients (t statistics in parentheses) | | | |
| | Number of Chronic Conditions | | Employment Status | |
	Zero Chronic Conditions	Some Chronic Conditions	Working Adults	Nonworking Adults
RAD	.143	.415	.393	.301
	(2.34)	(4.12)	(2.75)	(4.08)
CONDS	——	2.82	2.51	3.16
	——	(6.03)	(7.36)	(11.26)
AGE LT 15	.473	1.06	——	——
	(1.18)	(0.64)	——	——
AGE 45–64	.801	2.05	.546	1.71
	(2.07)	(1.52)	(0.73)	(1.42)
AGE 65+	2.62	3.33	3.32	2.37
	(4.91)	(2.10)	(2.53)	(1.95)
SEX	.243	.587	.581	1.176
	(0.85)	(0.65)	(0.77)	(1.46)
F 15–44	1.44	1.89	1.48	.821
	(3.17)	(1.18)	(1.39)	(0.66)
FAMSZ	−.064	.059	−.053	.195
	(0.82)	(0.20)	(−0.08)	(0.87)
WORKING	−.153	−1.080	——	——
	(0.52)	(−1.20)	——	——
NOINS	−.429	−1.94	.360	−.869
	(−1.39)	(1.76)	(0.44)	(−1.06)
FAMINC	−.00002	.00023	.0001	−.00001
	(1.07)	(2.70)	(1.81)	(−0.17)
GP/MD	−4.41	−2.61	−3.21	−3.21
	(−0.86)	(−0.15)	(−0.26)	(−0.24)
SURG/MD	−12.40	−10.51	8.23	−29.11
	(−1.17)	(−0.30)	(−0.33)	(−1.07)
POPDENS	.016	.018	.014	.019
	(0.93)	(0.97)	(0.81)	(1.14)
MDFEE	−.329	−1.35	−1.05	−.889
	(1.36)	(−1.54)	(−1.62)	(−1.38)
HOSCOST	.007	−.105	−.057	−.006
	(0.47)	(−2.22)	(−1.62)	(−0.18)
BEDS*	.775	−19.45	−16.29	−2.95
	(0.26)	(−2.11)	(−2.37)	(−0.41)
HBMD*	−13.78	31.09	−9.66	24.31
	(−1.49)	(1.01)	(−0.43)	(1.05)
OBMD*	21.48	91.89	43.83	52.82
	(1.92)	(2.53)	(1.68)	(1.82)
Constant	7.31	21.33	15.20	13.00
	(0.21)	(1.67)	(1.42)	(1.30)
$\bar{R}^2$	.041	.088	.269	.187
n	2096	1365	1359	1171
Visits Per Capita	3.67	8.97	5.00	7.55

Table 5.5   **Physician Visits Regressions, Aggregated Samples: Persons with Some Physician Visits**
(OLS)

Independent Statistic Variable or	Regression Coefficients (t statistics in parentheses)			
	22 Largest SMSAs	Other SMSAs	Nonmetro-politan Areas	All Areas
RAD	.196	.219	.274	.231
	(7.36)	(8.95)	(11.1)	(16.0)
CONDS	1.58	2.01	1.47	1.70
	(24.9)	(30.4)	(24.1)	(46.0)
AGE LT 15	.505	−.033	−.057	.128
	(2.64)	(−0.16)	(−0.29)	(1.11)
AGE 45–64	.704	.786	.737	.729
	(3.75)	(4.01)	(2.89)	(6.55)
AGE 65+	1.05	1.73	1.03	1.30
	(3.89)	(6.18)	(3.89)	(8.23)
SEX	.068	.172	−.004	.085
	(0.49)	(1.16)	(−0.03)	(1.07)
F 15–44	1.29	1.35	1.10	1.25
	(6.17)	(6.00)	(5.14)	(9.94)
FAMSZ	−.163	−.089	−.125	−.128
	(−5.73)	(−2.69)	(−3.93)	(−6.82)
WORKING	−.601	−.724	−.763	−.711
	(−4.36)	(−4.92)	(−5.49)	(−8.64)
NOINS	.269	−.166	−.096	.002
	(1.45)	(−0.87)	(−0.59)	(0.02)
FAMINC	.0006	−.002	−.0003	−.0007
	(0.63)	(−2.17)	(−0.26)	(−1.18)
GP/MD	.164	−2.74	.301	−.049
	(0.15)	(−1.19)	(0.49)	(−0.09)
SURG/MD	−4.05	−14.13	−1.50	−2.34
	(−1.82)	(−2.08)	(−1.39)	(−2.41)
POPDENS	−.033	.013	.100	.0005
	(−2.37)	(1.50)	(2.60)	(0.11)
MDFEE	.101	−.051	−.019	.063
	(2.90)	(−0.67)	(−0.50)	(2.63)
HOSCOST	−.004	−.004	.016	.007
	(−0.86)	(−0.63)	(3.17)	(2.27)
BEDS*	−1.37	−2.66	.128	−.267
	(−2.25)	(−2.31)	(0.39)	(−0.97)
HBMD*	−.540	−3.20	−.275	−1.73
	(−0.19)	(−0.71)	(−0.16)	(−1.33)
OBMD*	.700	.293	.981	1.42
	(0.22)	(0.05)	(1.10)	(1.66)
MIDED	−.027	.010	.008	−.018
	(−0.20)	(0.06)	(0.05)	(−0.21)
LOED	.088	.263	.035	.120
	(0.57)	(1.47)	(0.22)	(1.27)
SMMET	——	——	——	−.081
	——	——	——	(−0.20)

Table 5.5—*continued*

| Independent Statistic Variable or | Regression Coefficients (*t* statistics in parentheses) | | | |
	22 Largest SMSAs	Other SMSAs	Nonmetropolitan Areas	All Areas
RURAL	——	——	——	−.112
	——	——	——	(−0.67)
Constant	4.68	10.39	2.79	3.11
	(3.36)	(3.53)	(3.65)	(4.92)
$\bar{R}^2$	.113	.147	.129	.131
n	9736	11194	9427	30357

such a procedure prohibitively costly. Dummy variables for education of head and/or location were included in the regressions.

As indicated in table 5.5, physician stock has a positive but statistically insignificant effect in each of the three location subsamples even when all education groups are combined. When data are combined for all variables and all education levels, one does find that the coefficient on OBMD* is positive and significant at the 90% level. Even here the coefficient is numerically quite small. With such a large sample, statistical significance is usually to be expected. Moreover, the F-tests described above suggest that it is not proper to combine the subsamples and constrain coefficients to be equal across subsamples. Accordingly, it seems appropriate to conclude that a positive availability effect for persons with positive physician visits is difficult to detect, quite small in magnitude if it is found, and may be due only to specification error.[22]

For ambulatory visits, then, there appears to be little or no availability effect when other variables (including health measures) are properly controlled. It seems safe to conclude that, for the general population, the availability effect in ambulatory care can safely be ignored.

6   Hospital Beds, Hospital-oriented Physicians, and Hospital Use

In the previous chapter, I identified some effects on use of physicians' own services which may be caused by physician availability. Some kinds of physicians' services, such as surgical treatment, almost surely imply additional use of hospital facilities as well. In this chapter, I wish to investigate more deeply the determinants of hospital use, and of those physicians' services provided in connection with hospitalization, especially with regard to the relationship between the availability of hospital and physician inputs and hospital use.

The Relationship between Hospital Inputs and Use

There seems to be little a priori reason to expect that the availability of hospital inputs should lead to physician creation of demand for hospital care, and physicians seem to be the only group with the ability to create demand for hospital admissions. That is, there is no obvious reason why the mere availability of hospital inputs should lead a physician to try to affect patients' demand for medical care. If hospital inputs can be obtained at some vector of prices, the level of those inputs that would be chosen by a real-income-maximizing group of physicians will be based on the output to be produced and the relative prices (net of insurance) of hospital and other inputs. But this choice of inputs is simply the derived demand for inputs—it is determined by the demand for final output. It does not in any way determine that demand. The only connection between inputs and final output is through the effect of input prices on the quantities of inputs chosen, and on the consequent effect of those input costs on the price of final output. In this sense, the level of hospital inputs is wholly endogenous, and the availability or quantity of such inputs would not affect use in a casual sense. If hospital inputs are wholly endogenous, the quantities of those inputs should not affect the provision of information or any other way of shifting demand.

There are, however, reasons to suppose that the quantity of hospital inputs may not always be set at the level which physicians would demand. The most likely outcome is that the level of inputs will be low relative to what physicians would demand, so that excess demand will be observed. There are three possible causes of such an outcome. First, even if the hospital is run in the interests of physicians, there may be limitations on the hospital's ability to raise equity capital, which may in turn restrict its ability to provide physical or working capital. The number of donations to the hospital may have a direct influence on its capital stock, and may also affect the terms at which it can borrow. Second, the hospital's administration or trustees may not want to provide the inputs physicians and patients desire. It is an open empirical question whether the hospital's administration has the power to implement its desires, or, if it does, how one might characterize its preference function. But it is surely possible that it may choose not to provide inputs which physicians want, so that there will be excess demand. (Alternatively, the hospital may desire to provide facilities that patients and physicians do not want.) Finally, since demand for hospital services is stochastic, there will almost surely be temporary periods of excess demand (or excess supply) at the profit-maximizing level of inputs or even at other higher input levels. The self-limiting nature of many illnesses, or the possibility of substitution of ambulatory care for inpatient care, may turn such temporary shortages into permanent reductions in demand.

It is also possible that donations may be so large that the hospital has more capital than physicians would have desired if the opportunity cost of the capital had had to be covered by hospital charges. Such excess capital is, in the physicians' view, equivalent to donation of the implicit interest. It would, nevertheless, be expected to be put to use. In this sense, if the marginal unit of capital is raised from donations, actual capital stock may be treated as exogenous.

In what follows I will consider each of these three possible reasons for an availability effect for hospital care. The goal will be to see what they imply about the possible existence and causes of that effect. For purposes of present discussion, the supply of physicians will be taken to be exogenous.

Permanent Excess Demand

Suppose that hospitals are restricted in their ability to add beds, even though physicians acting as perfect agents would demand those beds for patients with some level of insurance coverage. Since the hospital must price approximately at average costs, there is no direct way in which the hospital price can be raised to ration demand. Feldstein has suggested that, in such circumstances, the physician will be under pressure to share capacity with others.[1] While this may be so, some form of nonprice rationing would obviously have to be used even in the absence of explicit pressure. Conversely, were there no excess demand, bed availability should not have a direct effect on the physician's desire to use beds or on the advice he gives to patients. The physician who is a perfect agent will only want to ration care if there is excess demand. He may try to keep "his" beds free in order to take care of an unexpected case; if the number of beds increases, he can admit more patients and still maintain the same safety margin. It is this excess demand, not the pressure on physicians, which is likely to be the ultimate cause of an availability effect. Any pressure on physicians, implicit or explicit, is only a manifestation of excess demand already present.

In the longer run, Feldstein describes a process of hospital price adjustment to excess demand that comes about through increases in the costliness, input intensity, and the quality of hospital care. What he ignores, and what may be critical, is the role played by physicians and *their* prices for services they provide in connection with inpatient care. Feldstein does provide a discussion of physician ambulatory services. As he suggests, these services may well be substitutes for hospitalization, and the conventional opinion is that there is a "shortage" of such primary care services. In such a case, the quantity supplied of such services, i.e., the position of the supply constraint, would indeed be more relevant than the price in determining actual use. The situation is more complicated if some observations display excess demand and some do not. Then prices may be relevant as well, although the precise econometric specification of the relationship is unclear.

But the point that Feldstein omits is that many physician services are complementary to hospital use. In the case in which the demand-for-admissions function can be written $Q_H = Q(P_M + P_H)$, where P_M is the physician's user (net of insurance) price (e.g., the uncovered portion of the surgeon's fee) and P_H is the hospital's user price, there is obviously a very strong form of complementarity. It implies not only that $\partial Q_H/\partial P_M < 0$, but that $\partial Q_H/\partial P_M = \partial Q_H/\partial P_H$.

Such strong complementarity would have important implications for the existence of permanent and continuous excess demand for hospital services. If there is no excess demand for hospital-oriented physician services such as surgery (which almost surely is the case), there can be no excess demand for hospital services either. Suppose demand and supply of hospital admissions are equated (given insurance coverage) at some set of prices $\bar{P}_M$, $\bar{P}_H$. Now let P_H be depressed below $\bar{P}_H$, to P_H', but with no corresponding increase in supply. Excess demand for hospital services will occur. Hospitals may choose not to raise their prices.

But this excess demand can also be eliminated by a rise in the price of physicians' services to P_M' so that $P_M' + P_H' = \bar{P}_M + \bar{P}_H$. If physicians' prices are sufficiently flexible upward, even a "shortage" of hospital beds need not lead to permanent excess demand.

Feldstein's explanation is that excess demand is gradually reduced as hospitals raise their prices and costs by shifting to higher "quality" care. The alternative explanation here is that at least part of the price rise occurs as increased physicians' fees. With the definition of what constitutes a physician's service and what constitutes a unit of hospital output fixed, there appears to be no alternative to this form of strict complementarity. As long as hospitalization requires fixed proportions of both hospital and physicians' services, such an explanation will be the appropriate one. Feldstein's explanation of how equilibrium is achieved in the market for hospital care may be seriously misleading.

Is there any sense in which a rise in the user price of hospital service would not have an effect on the demand for hospital services equal to that of a similar rise in the price of physicians' services? To the extent that the ratio of hospital to physician inputs can be varied, such a difference is surely possible. A decline in the user price of a day of stay, e.g., the room rate, will increase the demand for hospital admissions, but it will also lead to an increase in desired length of stay. Physicians' charges typically do not vary with length of stay or with other amenities. However, even here, since the same input (beds) is used to produce both admissions and days of stay, there cannot be an excess demand for beds. The supply of beds can be rationed by altering the number of admissions as well as by altering length of stay. Indeed, if physicians collectively can exert some control, one would expect them to favor a stay-intensive "bed rationing" policy, one which concentrates on shortening stays, rather than on an admissions-intensive policy, precisely because physician income depends more on admissions than length of stay.

The above discussion suggests that when beds are in short supply, physician prices will be higher, and it suggests that hospital prices alone may give an adequate explanation of hospital demand only if user prices P_M and P_H are highly correlated. Such correlation is probably present in general; whatever the case with gross prices, hospital insurance coverage and insurance for physicians' services in hospital are highly correlated (as one would expect, since they are really the "same" insurance). What is critical, of course, is whether physician prices are sufficiently flexible upwards so that they will clear the market. At this point, we do not know whether they are or not.

Another less likely possibility is that there may be excess supplies of beds. This would generally result from incorrect planning, from demand shifts, or from overly generous public subsidies or private donations.

From the viewpoint of the hospital's administration or trustees, using those empty beds would probably be desirable. But there are no direct incentives to physicians to have them filled, no direct physician gain from admitting an additional patient whom the physician would not have wished to admit in the absence of empty beds. The hospital's financial condition can, however, have some *indirect* effects on physician decisions. If filling an empty bed reduces a deficit that threatens hospital survival, physicians collectively may agree to shift or tailor patient demand to fill empty facilities.

If the hospital is not in such difficulties, filling empty beds may still mean additional hospital profits (or smaller losses). Whether or not filling empty beds increases hospital profits depends on how the hospital is paid. If insurance pays wholly on the basis of costs, additional filled beds may please the administrator who values output, but they do not add to profits as long as incremental insurance reimbursement exactly equals incremental cost. If reimbursement exceeds marginal costs, and if filling of empty beds does not seriously affect the hospital's ability to handle peaks in demands, then physicians might be willing to create some additional demand if *they* can benefit in some way from the hospital's increased flow of profits.

One avenue of benefit would be the use of profits from filled beds to subsidize other outputs the hospital produces. Since the amount the physician can collect for the physician-hospital joint product increases as the hospital price is reduced, such a strategy would be a way of transferring the hospital's profits to physicians. Since the utility loss to the physician from increasing demand above what he would have chosen in the absence of excess beds is initially very small, and since the gain to him from hospital profits is positive, some demand creation would make him better off. A second strategy is for the hospital to use the additional profits for capital improvements which enhance physician income or utility. This strategy would be more likely to be chosen if the hospital could not transfer its profits directly to physicians. If it could transfer profits, the hospital which happens to have earned profits would make investments it would not have made in the absence of funds from profits only if there were restrictions on its ability to borrow. Note that, in all cases, the incentive to increase hospital demand must be imposed *collectively* on physicians. Otherwise, each individual physician would prefer to ride free; he would prefer to maintain his own level of accuracy while gaining from the hospital profits generated by other physicians' demand creation efforts.

Thus it is theoretically possible for an excess supply of beds to induce physicians to engage in more information manipulation, although the connection between an individual physician's reduction in accuracy and his income is not nearly so direct as for physicians' services themselves. Whether or not bed-availability effects actually do differ across education-information groups provides a test of the coincidence between theoretical possibility and reality.

Physicians and Hospital Administrators

If permanent excess demand does not necessarily arise from supply side restrictions, can it arise because hospital administrators refuse to provide beds that physicians and patients both demand and are willing to pay for through insurance? Such an event surely seems implausible. It is more likely that hospital administrators will desire *more* output than do physicians. Indeed, the supply of beds might be expected to be restricted by a physician cartel, but such restrictions would probably be opposed by individual hospital administrators.

Even empty beds may satisfy the administrator's desire for a large plant to manage. Of course, empty beds may also embarrass him or cause him financial difficulties.

Stochastic Demand

A more likely explanation for excess demand for hospital beds than any of those discussed so far is provided by the stochastic nature of demand. There can be *temporary* excess demand. The reason is simple: it will not ordinarily be desirable to build a hospital of such a size that there will never be excess demand, and it is impossible to vary prices to eliminate temporary shortages. Beyond some point, beds cannot be substituted for other inputs, or vice versa, to permit the hospital to deal with all levels of demand. So there will sometimes be excess demand; the level of total hospital demand will be inversely related to the probability of shortage, and directly related to bed supply. If the hospital is sometimes full, ambulatory care may be substituted, or the patient's condition may cure itself while he waits for a bed. Whatever the mechanism by which the choice is made, not all communities will end up with the same probability of shortage. Those communities in which the probability is smaller will, of course, have more use of hospitals. The possibility of temporary excess demand, therefore, provides a plausible explanation for an effect of hospital beds on hospital use.

When a hospital does happen to be full, there will be pressures on physicians to ration beds. One would expect that this rationing would have to be done on some collective basis, even if only implicitly. Physicians may even manipulate information to reduce the level of demand to hospital capacity. The critical point, however, is that physician behavior is solely a response to excess demand, and does not require a separate theory of demand creation. There may still be some differences between educational groups in the extent to which their demands can be affected by whatever form of nonprice rationing physicians choose, although there is no a priori reason to expect differences.

Physicians and Hospital Use

What might be the effect of physician availability on hospital use? For those physicians who primarily provide substitutes for inpatient care, such as general practitioners, use of hospital services might be expected to decrease with an increase in the absolute or relative number of such physicians (prices held constant), if there is an availability effect on the demand for ambulatory services. Where there is no such effect, only the relative prices of hospital substitutes would be relevant. With regard to hospital-oriented physicians who provide complementary inputs, such as surgical specialists, anything that increases the use of these physicians' inputs will also increase the use of the associated hospital inputs. It is generally agreed that there is an excess supply of many of these complementary physician inputs, especially general surgeons. An observed availability effect is therefore unlikely to arise from even temporary excess demand. If a physician availability effect occurs, it almost surely must come from information manipulation. For some other specialties, such as internal medicine, the prediction is ambiguous, since we do not know whether they are primarily producers of substitutes for or complements to hospital care.

If there is true demand creation, one should therefore look for an availability effect running from surgeon stock to use of surgeons' services in hospital. That such an effect exists has been suggested in the empirical literature, most strongly by Bunker, who found high rates of surgery matched by high rates of surgeons per capita in a comparison of the United States to England and Wales.[2] Lewis found that for some (but not all) surgical procedures there was a significant relationship between surgeon availability and surgery.[3] Wennberg and Gittelsohn also found this relationship, especially at the extremes of their small number of observations, but it seemed to break down at the level of individual surgical procedures.[4] This is perhaps not unexpected; there is no reason to suppose that demand creation, if it occurs, necessarily takes the same form everywhere.

Empirical Tests

The basic form and set of exogenous variables for the hospital demand equations that are presented in the next section are the same as for the physician visit equations in chapter 5. Independent variables are defined in the same way. Since federal hospital beds are not included in the measure of BEDS*, persons with episodes in federal hospitals were dropped from this sample, reducing the sample size slightly from that used in chapter 5.

Because any effect of beds on use will probably not come from information manipulation, there is no a priori expectation that there will be a difference between education-information groups in the coefficients measuring the effects of bed availability on either length of stay or admissions. If education somehow proxied time cost, and given suitable differences in the form of the demand function, some differences might emerge, but it would be difficult to predict them a priori. Indeed, the effect of stochastic excess demand may be too small to detect, especially if the occupancy rate is low enough that the hospital is rarely full.

Length of stay should depend primarily upon hospital and patient variables, but not directly on physician availability or price. One caveat is, however, suggested by the results in chapter 3. If a larger number of physicians per capita means more physician time spent at the hospital, this additional input may reduce length of stay. Since we have no accurate measure of the price of such an input, but only an overall index of physician medical or surgical fees, it is possible that in those areas where there are relatively many physicians and in which patients demand larger amounts of physician inputs per day of stay, stays may be shorter. Such an inverse relationship between physicians per capita and stay may be telling us more about production technology than demand.

Physicians would be most likely to have a demand-creation effect in the case of those hospital admissions in which surgery is performed. The surgically treated episode measures both the output which is of concern to the surgeon—the surgical procedure he performs—and the use by the patient of complementary hospital inputs. The relevant measure of availability here would be surgical specialists per capita. The fraction of physicians who are G.P.'s is also included in order to measure, in a crude way, the possibilities for substitution of nonsurgical for surgical forms of treatment. The physician price variable for surgically treated episodes (MDFEE) is a weighted average (over general practitioners and specialists) of the 1973 Medicare prevailing charge for hernia repair. For total hospital episodes, the followup office visit fee is used as a general index of physician fee levels. Finally, the number of hospital-based physicians per capita is included to take account of possible substitutes for surgical specialists. Ideally, we would like to have known the fraction of hospital-based physicians who are surgical specialists, but this fraction should be highly correlated with the total.

Results

Table 6.1 indicates the results for tobit and OLS regressions using hospital admissions as the dependent variable. While some persons had

Table 6.1 Annual Hospital Episodes Regressions, All Episodes (Tobit and OLS Procedures)

Regression Coefficients (t statistics in parentheses)

Independent Variable or Statistic	22 Largest SMSAs				Other SMSAs				Nonmetropolitan Areas			
	Low Head Education		High Head Education		Low Head Education		Education High Head		Low Head Education		High Head Education	
	Tobit	OLS	Tobit	OLS	Tobit	OLS	Tobit	OLS	Tobit	OLS	Tobit	OLS
RAD	.108 (6.47)	.025 (10.2)	.157 (5.76)	.037 (10.4)	.115 (5.91)	.024 (8.21)	.138 (5.84)	.039 (9.00)	.135 (7.96)	.039 (12.7)	.095 (3.54)	.021 (5.42)
CONDS	.431 (7.93)	.059 (8.87)	.246 (2.95)	.013 (1.54)	.427 (7.10)	.054 (7.17)	.480 (7.38)	.070 (7.80)	.436 (8.68)	.328 (8.33)	.064 (5.12)	.039 (4.93)
AGE LT 15	−.308 (−1.46)	−.041 (−2.02)	−.603 (−2.13)	−.073 (−3.02)	−.591 (−2.52)	−.060 (−2.62)	.040 (.19)	−.015 (−0.64)	−.441 (−2.11)	−.053 (−2.18)	−.202 (−0.88)	−.050 (−2.11)
AGE 45–64	.241 (1.29)	.004 (0.22)	.293 (1.05)	.022 (0.95)	.095 (0.45)	.006 (0.30)	.555 (2.62)	.043 (2.31)	.523 (2.87)	.049 (2.23)	.809 (3.67)	.070 (3.10)
AGE 65+	.425 (1.90)	.030 (1.28)	.733 (1.95)	.099 (2.73)	.198 (0.76)	.015 (0.53)	.954 (3.53)	.150 (3.72)	.456 (2.03)	.058 (1.95)	.656 (2.19)	.641 (1.90)
SEX	−.066 (−0.50)	−.003 (−0.22)	−.118 (−0.53)	−.012 (−0.63)	.178 (1.16)	.014 (0.91)	−.152 (−.97)	−.019 (−1.04)	−.122 (−0.93)	−.017 (−1.05)	−.273 (−1.66)	−.024 (−1.44)
F 15–44	.850 (3.93)	.070 (3.19)	1.175 (3.84)	.106 (3.96)	.399 (1.63)	.036 (1.44)	1.24 (5.36)	.152 (5.72)	1.11 (5.22)	.134 (4.95)	1.277 (5.01)	.111 (4.37)
FAMSZ	.0005 (0.02)	−.0004 (−0.11)	.037 (0.86)	.004 (0.90)	.011 (0.31)	.001 (0.37)	−.044 (−1.30)	−.003 (−0.78)	−.014 (−0.48)	−.001 (−0.28)	−.003 (−0.07)	−.005 (−0.13)
WORKING	−.263 (−2.07)	−.032 (−2.29)	−.572 (−3.04)	−.067 (−3.61)	−.307 (−2.15)	−.034 (−2.19)	−.342 (−2.35)	−.054 (−2.82)	−.324 (−2.62)	−.058 (−3.46)	−.521 (−3.42)	−.079 (−4.46)
NOINS	.361 (2.38)	−.021 (−1.46)	.072 (0.26)	−.009 (−0.37)	.261 (1.59)	−.207 (1.27)	—	—	.330 (2.47)	−.039 (2.46)	—	—
FAMINC	−.00004 (−0.04)	.00002 (0.17)	−.0004 (−0.40)	−.0 (−0.02)	.001 (0.68)	.0001 (0.83)	.0004 (0.48)	−.0 (−0.02)	.003 (2.15)	.0004 (2.18)	−.0005 (−0.53)	−.0001 (0.53)
GP/MD	−4.13 (−1.74)	−.506 (−2.06)	−6.240 (−2.35)	−.428 (−1.73)	1.18 (0.89)	.126 (0.96)	1.61 (1.24)	.201 (1.34)	.503 (0.08)	.038 (0.49)	.161 (0.23)	.014 (0.19)

Table 6.1—*continued*

Regression Coefficients (*t* statistics in parentheses)

Independent Variable or Statistic	22 Largest SMSAs				Other SMSAs				Nonmetropolitan Areas			
	Low Head Education		High Head Education		Low Head Education		Education High Head		Low Head Education		High Head Education	
	Tobit	OLS	Tobit	OLS	Tobit	OLS	Tobit	OLS	Tobit	OLS	Tobit	OLS
SURG/MD	−7.35	−.738	−10.56	−.823	4.09	.410	4.82	.503	.372	.129	−1.297	−.117
	(−1.45)	(−1.43)	(−1.75)	(−1.49)	(1.61)	(1.55)	(1.91)	(1.90)	(0.35)	(0.96)	(−0.99)	(−0.83)
POPDENS	.002	.0002	.002	−.0004	.017	.002	−.007	−.0005	.078	.018	−.007	.004
	(0.26)	(0.42)	(0.17)	(−0.03)	(1.06)	(0.97)	(−0.50)	(−0.33)	(2.20)	(2.09)	(−0.17)	(0.11)
MDFEE	−.161	−.019	−.063	−.002	−.013	−.001	.042	−.005	−.065	−.005	.035	.003
	(−2.31)	(−2.54)	(−0.61)	(−0.15)	(−0.34)	(−0.03)	(1.26)	(−1.50)	(−1.45)	(0.99)	(0.98)	(0.73)
HOSCOST	.008	—	.002	—	.0003	−.0003	.008	.0007	−.003	−.0004	.003	.0005
	(1.30)		(0.22)		(−0.04)	(−0.45)	(1.55)	(−1.50)	(−0.57)	(−0.52)	(0.62)	(0.80)
BEDS*	1.39	.104	.965	.039	.926	.062	.729	.102	.264	.015	1.152	.133
	(1.21)	(0.83)	(0.69)	(0.30)	(1.43)	(0.88)	(1.12)	(1.50)	(0.79)	(0.34)	(3.37)	(3.60)
HBMD*	−1.44	−.298	−10.67	−.105	.713	.004	−1.36	−.170	−2.07	−.178	−2.65	−.309
	(−0.35)	(−0.68)	(−1.75)	(−1.99)	(0.70)	(0.01)	(−0.93)	(−0.55)	(−1.14)	(−0.84)	(−1.68)	(−1.77)
OBMD*	−2.26	−.418	−8.87	−1.20	−1.82	−.085	.759	.172	1.79	.151	−.69	−.051
	(−0.47)	(−0.82)	(−1.39)	(−2.01)	(−0.54)	(−0.21)	(0.27)	(0.42)	(1.54)	(0.87)	(−0.85)	(−0.67)
Constant	.286	.499	3.01	.572	−5.29	−.130	−6.49	−.133	−3.27	.011	−3.25	.048
	(0.09)	(1.57)	(0.92)	(1.88)	(−3.26)	(−0.76)	(−4.26)	(−1.93)	(−4.12)	(0.11)	(−3.97)	(0.55)
$\bar{R}^2$ or significance of Chi-square statistic	.000	.075	.000	.082	.000	.060	.000	.082	.000	.098	.000	.057
n	4985	4985	2683	2683	3811	3811	3942	3942	4639	4639	3155	3155
F statistic for hypothesis of inequality of regression coefficients	1.95				1.56				1.51			

$F_{.01}$ (19, large *n*) = 1.88
$F_{.05}$ (19, large *n*) = 1.57

NOTE: Means and standard deviations are shown in appendix table 1.

multiple episodes, many had zero, and about 80% of those with some admissions had just one admission.

Admissions Rates

The effect of beds on hospital admissions per year is positive in all regressions, but is significant only for high education families in rural areas. F-tests indicate that the hypothesis of equality of the sets of regression coefficients across the education subsamples cannot be rejected at the 95% level for the rural and other metropolitan samples. The sets of coefficients are different for the large urban sample, but in that sample the coefficients on BEDS* do not differ significantly.[5] The results are therefore consistent with the hypothesis that an effect of availability of beds on use, if observed, should not be attributed to demand creation or information manipulation. Physician variables (OBMD* and HBMD*) more frequently have a negative than a positive effect on use, but are significant only for the high education persons in large cities in the OLS regression. As discussed in chapter 5, physician variables for this subsample have a significant negative effect on the use of ambulatory physicians' services as well.

Physician and hospital prices frequently have a negative effect on use, as does the absence of insurance coverage, but these variables are significant only for a few of the subsamples. The composition of the physician stock (GP/MD and SURG/MD) has no consistent effect on use of hospitals. Finally, variables measuring health status, work status, age, and female of childbearing age are almost always significantly related to use in the expected directions.

To summarize: availability variables generally have little consistent or significant effect on admission rates in these educational subgroups. The question of the effect of availability variables on total hospital admissions will be discussed in more detail below. These results for the subgroups do suggest, however, that the primary determinant of use is the health status of individuals, *not* the availability of beds or physicians.

Length of Stay

The results for length of stay, shown in table 6.2, display a similar pattern. Stay is more frequently positively related to beds, but the effect is small and is significant only for the high education subgroup in smaller metropolitan areas. Stay tends to be shorter where physicians are more plentiful, perhaps because more physicians can monitor their hospitalized patients more closely. Gross prices and physician stock specialty composition are unrelated to length of stay, while the existence of insurance coverage has negative but inconsistent effects.

Patient characteristics variables have the expected effects on stay, although the effects of health status variables are estimated less pre-

Table 6.2   **Average Length of Stay Regressions, All Episodes**
(OLS)

	22 Largest SMSAs		Other SMSAs		Nonmetropolitan Areas	
Independent Variable or Statistic	Low Head Education Low Head	High Head Education High Head	Low Head Education Low Head	High Head Education High Head	Low Head Education Low Head	High Head Education High Head
RAD	.107	−.306	.208	−.117	.254	.168
	(0.91)	(−1.40)	(0.28)	(−0.60)	(3.34)	(1.76)
CONDS	1.02	1.81	.757	−.42	.451	.035
	(2.17)	(2.02)	(0.80)	(0.64)	(1.70)	(0.07)
AGE LT 15	−6.74	−4.36	−2.29	−9.18	−2.02	−1.53
	(3.13)	(−1.28)	(−0.49)	(−2.99)	(−1.40)	(−0.82)
AGE 45–64	1.71	4.69	6.05	−1.26	2.50	2.26
	(0.86)	(1.29)	(1.51)	(0.45)	(2.08)	(1.26)
AGE 65+	−.151	1.80	12.92	4.76	2.34	5.76
	(−0.06)	(0.43)	(2.73)	(1.43)	(1.63)	(2.56)
SEX	−1.71	−3.61	−6.08	4.09	−1.70	−1.88
	(−1.36)	(−1.28)	(−2.18)	(2.02)	(−2.12)	(−1.42)
F 15–44	−2.81	−1.10	1.85	−10.6	−.614	.436
	(−1.33)	(−0.29)	(0.41)	(−3.38)	(−0.44)	(0.22)
FAMSZ	.170	−.848	.457	.232	.154	−.274
	(0.53)	(−1.66)	(0.64)	(.50)	(0.86)	(0.89)
WORKING	−2.93	−2.20	.378	−3.82	−.910	−1.75
	(2.72)	(−1.00)	(0.15)	(−2.04)	(−1.21)	(−1.54)
NOINS	4.41	5.72	−6.49	——	.909	——
	(2.99)	(1.95)	(−2.14)	——	(−1.08)	——
FAMINC	.004	−.002	.013	.004	−.0006	.007
	(0.42)	(−0.14)	(0.53)	(0.44)	(−0.07)	(1.03)
GP/MD	25.5	2.37	11.7	−24.20	.120	5.18
	(1.06)	(0.11)	(0.46)	(−1.43)	(0.03)	(0.97)
SURG/MD	29.1	−18.6	5.71	−38.2	1.74	1.38
	(0.54)	(0.28)	(0.12)	(−1.19)	(0.27)	(0.14)
POPDENS	−.026	.155	−.421	−.137	−.043	−.038
	(−0.18)	(1.02)	(−1.26)	(−0.70)	(−0.23)	(−0.11)
MDFEE	.410	.015	.692	1.24	−0.11	.216
	(0.62)	(0.06)	(0.83)	(3.15)	(−0.40)	(0.80)
HOSCOST	.024	.046	−.134	−.083	−.012	.001
	(0.39)	(0.48)	(−1.17)	(−1.22)	(−0.43)	(0.22)
BEDS*	9.88	−8.19	−1.77	20.8	−2.77	1.20
	(0.85)	(−0.50)	(−0.14)	(2.36)	(−1.32)	(0.45)
HBMD*	77.7	−38.1	95.9	−.959	6.48	4.01
	(1.93)	(0.43)	(1.90)	(−0.02)	(0.53)	(0.33)
OBMD*	−38.1	−110.5	−81.9	−51.5	1.90	1.73
	(−0.80)	(1.63)	(−1.13)	(−1.2)	(0.32)	(0.24)
Constant	−11.44	2.12	17.33	21.8	6.68	.902
	(−0.36)	(0.04)	(0.54)	(1.1)	(1.37)	(0.13)
$\bar{R}^2$	.092	.064	.043	.123	.100	.064

Regression Coefficients (t statistics in parentheses)

Table 6.2—*continued*

	Regression Coefficients (*t* statistics in parentheses)					
	22 Largest SMSAs		Other SMSAs		Nonmetropolitan Areas	
Independent Variable or Statistic	Low Head Education	High Head Education	Low Head Education	High Head Education	Low Head Education	High Head Education
n	496	218	375	363	529	295
F statistic for hypothesis of inequality of regression coefficients	0.99		1.58		0.08	
F .05 (19, large *n*) = 1.57						

NOTE: Means and standard deviations are shown in appendix table 3.

cisely than in the other regressions. Children, women, and persons who are working tend to have shorter stays, and older persons longer ones.

Surgically Treated Hospital Episodes

It is widely believed that there is an "excess" of surgical specialists. While this definition is usually based on technical notions of how much work a surgeon can do, rather than on behavioral notions of how much work the surgeon is willing to do, one can interpret it as suggesting that there is an excess supply of surgeons' services. It will therefore be desirable to see whether the amount of in-hospital surgery (measured by the number of surgically treated hospital episodes, other than those for delivery) is related, *ceteris paribus*, to the stock of surgical specialists available to perform surgery.

Table 6.3 indicates the results of regressions of surgically treated hospital episodes using the same set of variables as before, except that SURG/MD has been deleted and surgical specialists per capita (SURG*) has been substituted for office based physicians per capita. The results for surgical episodes are similar to those obtained in the analysis of all hospital episodes. Hospital beds tend to be related positively to use, but the effect is not very strong nor is it measured very precisely; as in the case of all hospital episodes, it is significant only for high education families in rural areas. Physician stock specialty composition and gross price are not strongly related to the use of surgery. What is perhaps most striking is the finding that the number of surgical specialists per capita is not significantly related to the amount of surgery for any of the education-location subgroups. Indeed, the coefficient on this variable is negative in five out of six regressions. While these insignificant effects

Table 6.3 Surgically Treated Hospital Episode Regressions Except Episodes for Normal Delivery: Tobit and OLS Procedures

Regression Coefficients (t statistics in parentheses)

Independent Variable or Statistic	22 Largest SMSAs				Other SMSAs				Nonmetropolitan Areas			
	Low Head Education		High Head Education		Low Head Education		High Head Education		Low Head Education		High Head Education	
	Tobit	OLS	Tobit	OLS	Tobit	OLS	Tobit	OLS	Tobit	OLS	Tobit	OLS
RAD	.111 (5.55)	.013 (8.39)	.143 (4.47)	.016 (7.38)	.145 (6.40)	.018 (10.0)	.131 (4.28)	.017 (6.74)	.116 (5.54)	.015 (8.25)	.080 (2.22)	.010 (3.74)
CONDS	.330 (4.85)	.024 (5.49)	.325 (3.22)	.012 (2.37)	.245 (3.14)	.011 (2.19)	.494 (5.89)	.032 (6.26)	.348 (5.37)	.026 (5.71)	.374 (4.39)	.024 (4.46)
AGE LT 15	−.001 (−.01)	−.004 (−.29)	−.413 (−1.17)	−.017 (−1.18)	−.304 (−1.02)	−.013 (−.90)	−.062 (−.21)	−.005 (−.34)	−.475 (−1.79)	−.023 (−1.66)	−.021 (−.07)	−.008 (−.53)
AGE 45–64	.304 (1.32)	.008 (0.63)	−.332 (−.993)	−.008 (−0.62)	.127 (.47)	.007 (.53)	.398 (1.44)	.027 (1.96)	.216 (.94)	.009 (0.67)	.846 (2.93)	.049 (3.24)
AGE 65+	.349 (1.23)	.009 (0.62)	.331 (.713)	.027 (1.26)	.058 (.18)	.0004 (.61)	.413 (1.08)	.014 (0.70)	−.174 (−.58)	−.015 (−.87)	.637 (1.58)	.033 (1.49)
SEX	−.041 (−.25)	−.0004 (0.05)	.197 (−.714)	.004 (0.33)	.331 (1.74)	.013 (1.34)	−.193 (−0.91)	−.012 (−1.17)	.127 (.73)	.006 (.64)	−.189 (−.88)	−.009 (−0.76)
F 15–44	.582 (2.14)	.023 (1.56)	.376 (.989)	.024 (1.53)	.075 (.24)	.007 (0.46)	.518 (1.66)	.021 (1.33)	.337 (1.23)	.020 (1.30)	.521 (1.55)	.018 (1.04)
FAMSZ	.003 (.08)	−.0005 (−.24)	−.035 (−.625)	−.002 (−.71)	−.011 (−.24)	−.001 (−.53)	−.018 (−.38)	−.002 (−.69)	.008 (.21)	−.0002 (−.08)	−.007 (−.13)	−.0006 (−.21)
WORKING	.002 (.01)	.0009 (0.95)	−.209 (−.853)	−.010 (−.96)	−.093 (−.51)	−.0006 (−.06)	−.249 (−1.21)	−.017 (−1.58)	−.063 (−.39)	−.006 (−.65)	−.280 (−1.29)	−.022 (−1.91)
NOINS	.378 (1.99)	−.009 (−.99)	−.313 (−.972)	.016 (1.16)	.397 (1.84)	−.018 (1.76)	—	—	.545 (2.97)	−.023 (−2.65)	—	—
FAMINC	.0002 (.143)	.00 (0.41)	.00006 (0.06)	.00 (0.06)	.0008 (0.50)	.0001 (0.62)	.002 (1.79)	.00009 (1.61)	.004 (2.83)	.0003 (2.93)	.001 (1.26)	.00007 (1.17)
GP/MD	−.498 (−.329)	−.062 (−.72)	−.649 (−.298)	−.074 (−.82)	−1.32 (−1.13)	−.035 (−.60)	−2.122 (−1.85)	−.086 (−1.53)	−.525 (−1.13)	−.024 (−.95)	.915 (1.95)	.043 (1.75)
POPDENS	.0004 (.044)	.0002 (0.40)	.008 (.571)	.0003 (0.47)	−.029 (−1.40)	−.0009 (−.81)	.006 (0.32)	.0007 (0.72)	.108 (2.63)	.009 (3.24)	−.045 (−.70)	−.002 (−.70)

Table 6.3—continued

Regression Coefficients (t statistics in parentheses)

Independent Variable or Statistic	22 Largest SMSAs				Other SMSAs				Nonmetropolitan Areas			
	Low Head Education		High Head Education		Low Head Education		High Head Education		Low Head Education		High Head Education	
	Tobit	OLS	Tobit	OLS	Tobit	OLS	Tobit	OLS	Tobit	OLS	Tobit	OLS
MDFEE	−.003 (−3.000)	−.008 (−1.89)	−.002 (−1.000)	−.003 (−.63)	.0009 (.39)	−.001 (−.44)	.002 (1.20)	.0008 (.35)	−.002 (.81)	−.003 (−.89)	−.00003 (−.02)	−.0001 (−.04)
HOSCOST	.007 (1.000)	.0006 (1.28)	−.011 (−1.100)	−.002 (−.47)	−.008 (−1.2)	−.0001 (−.33)	−.0001 (−.02)	.0001 (.29)	−.002 (−.26)	−.002 (−.36)	.008 (1.05)	.0004 (.94)
BEDS*	1.64 (1.106)	.094 (1.16)	−.251 (−.142)	−.030 (−.41)	.229 (.27)	.016 (.34)	.123 (.13)	.004 (.08)	.318 (.70)	.011 (.43)	1.01 (2.15)	.052 (2.12)
HBMD*	−3.11 (−.004)	.042 (.14)	−3.16 (−.420)	−.091 (−.29)	−4.62 (1.13)	−.208 (−.97)	−1.83 (−.37)	−.032 (−.16)	−1.98 (−.83)	−.071 (−.58)	−.97 (−.46)	−.006 (−.05)
SURG*	19.538 (.949)	.832 (.75)	15.296 (.513)	−.317 (−.27)	−15.151 (−1.17)	−.040 (−.05)	−2.025 (−.17)	−.039 (−.06)	−2.838 (−.43)	−.107 (−.31)	−1.770 (−.44)	−.090 (−.49)
Constant	−5.31 (−3.568)	−.001 (.02)	−2.17 (−1.198)	.130 (1.61)	−3.03 (−2.83)	.049 (.81)	−4.36 (−4.6)	.025 (.48)	−4.10 (−5.21)	.025 (.61)	−5.24 (−7.05)	−.025 (−.60)
R̄² or significance of Chi-square statistic	.000	.036	.000	.035	.000	.039	.000	.034	.000	.042	.000	.024
n	4985	4985	2693	2693	3811	3811	3942	3942	4639	4639	3155	3155
F statistic for hypothesis of inequality of regression coefficients			1.02				2.11				2.10	
F.01 (18, large n) = 1.88												

NOTE: Means and standard deviations are shown in appendix table 1.

could possibly be explained for persons living in rural areas by the fact that they may travel out of their primary sampling unit for care, very few of the persons in SMSAs are likely to leave the metropolitan area. In summary, the results do not differ across education subgroups, and are not even positive or significant. In view of these striking results (or nonresults), a more direct test of the existence of any availability effect for surgical services will be presented in the next section.

The effects of other independent variables on the use of surgery are similar to those in the overall hospital episodes regressions. Health status measures are strongly related to use: sicker people are more likely to have had surgery. Somewhat surprisingly, consumption of surgery tends to be highest, *ceteris paribus*, among the middle aged (45–64). There is a weak positive relationship between the frequency of surgery and females of childbearing age status, and a weak negative relationship with being employed. Insurance is fairly strongly related to the use of surgery for the lower education group, while family income is weakly related.

Availability Effects and the Use of Hospitals

The original hypothesis of the availability effect, often called Roemer's law, was derived from a study which found a positive relationship between the number of hospital beds and their use.[6] In a similar way, the notion that surgeons cause surgery is a strong point of health services research folklore, even though the results in the often-cited study by Lewis do not, in fact, provide very strong statistical support for the proposition.[7]

In the education-area subgroups investigated in this study, however, no such availability effects were found. F-tests shown in tables 6.1 to 6.3 indicate that, in many of the subsamples, it is preferable to permit the coefficients to differ by education subgroups. In principle, one should therefore test for the *overall* effect of any variable, such as BEDS* or SURG*, by including it interacting with the education dummies, and by interacting all other independent variables with those dummies. In practice, the large sample size makes such a procedure costly, and the results are often difficult to interpret in any case. As an alternative, we examined OLS regressions on data combined for all education groups within each area, as well as data aggregated over all areas. Dummies were introduced for education or location; no further interaction was attempted.

The results in table 6.4 do suggest that there is a weak effect of BEDS* on total admissions for the full sample (all education groups, all areas) even though the effect was not significant for the subsamples. Moreover, the magnitude of the effect is in any case quite small, with an elasticity of about 0.1. BEDS* has no overall effect on either length of stay or surgical admissions.

As before, we find that neither the surgeons per capita variable nor the other measures of physician stock are significant in any of the aggregated surgical episodes regressions. Physician stock and measures of the composition of physician stock likewise have no effects on total episodes or on length of stay. Physician availability does not belong in regressions describing hospital use.

An effect which does come through much more clearly in these aggregated samples is the effect of insurance on hospital use. Since almost all high education families have coverage, a no-insurance dummy was used to indicate only those low and middle education persons without coverage. For both total episodes and surgical episodes, there is a highly significant negative effect of lack of insurance coverage on use. The calculated admission rate for persons who lack insurance would be about 30 to 40% less than for persons with insurance. A somewhat surprising offset, however, is that persons with insurance tend to have significantly shorter stays than persons without insurance. The two effects nearly cancel out in terms of expected hospital days, although insurance coverage still probably has a positive effect on total expenditures.

Gross physician fees or hospital prices (which tend to be positively correlated) do not have a significant effect on total episodes, surgery, or length of stay. At a relatively low level of significance, there is a suggestion that high hospital prices reduce length of stay, while high surgical fees (especially in big cities) tend to discourage surgery. The results of these aggregate regressions are therefore roughly similar to those obtained from the disaggregated regressions. Availability effects on hospital use are small or nonexistent, and do not appear to arise from demand creation.

In particular, more surgeons do not mean more surgery. In contrast, a recent study by Fuchs, using the same data presented here but aggregating it into regional rates, presents the finding that surgeon availability is related to surgery rates, although the effect is relatively small (an elasticity of 0.3).[8] How can this finding be reconciled with those presented here?

There are two possibilities. First, this study has used many more personal characteristics, especially health status measures, than did Fuchs. While he did use 2SLS and treat surgeon stock as endogenous, possible correlation (whether causal or not) between health status variables and the variables used to predict surgeon stock could lead to the finding of a spurious effect.

Second, there is a potentially important group of consumers which was not included in this sample, but was included in the calculations of

Table 6.4   **Aggregated Sample Regressions: Hospital Episodes, Length of Stay, and Surgically Treated Episodes (OLS)**

Regression Coefficients (*t* statistics in parentheses)

Independent Variable or Statistic	All Episodes				Surgically Treated Episodes				Average Length of Stay			
	22 Large SMSAs	Other SMSAs	Non-metro Areas	All Areas	22 Large SMSAs	Other SMSAs	Non-metro Areas	All Areas	22 Large SMSAs	Other SMSAs	Non-metro Areas	All Areas
RAD	.028 (19.3)	.026 (14.3)	.034 (18.0)	.029 (29.8)	.015 (14.7)	.015 (12.7)	.014 (12.18)	.015 (23.0)	.125 (1.68)	.196 (1.78)	.211 (3.35)	.167 (3.51)
CONDS	.047 (12.6)	.046 (10.9)	.050 (11.4)	.048 (20.1)	.022 (8.63)	.019 (6.73)	.022 (8.32)	.021 (13.7)	1.15 (4.05)	.251 (0.64)	.392 (1.84)	.563 (3.31)
AGE LT 15	−.044 (−4.03)	−.036 (−3.03)	−.045 (−3.44)	−.042 (−6.13)	−.011 (−1.45)	−.010 (−1.24)	−.013 (−1.60)	−.011 (−2.51)	−5.96 (−4.78)	−3.34 (−2.01)	−2.89 (−2.94)	−4.21 (−5.56)
AGE 45–64	.033 (3.24)	.028 (2.44)	.047 (3.80)	.036 (5.50)	.014 (2.13)	.014 (1.81)	.020 (2.62)	.016 (3.76)	.071 (0.06)	2.70 (1.73)	1.70 (1.92)	1.26 (1.84)
AGE 65+	.036 (2.45)	.062 (3.75)	.060 (3.38)	.052 (5.46)	.007 (0.70)	.015 (1.31)	.006 (0.60)	.009 (1.46)	−.232 (−0.16)	8.02 (4.23)	4.62 (4.09)	4.07 (4.71)
SEX	−.014 (−1.75)	.005 (0.56)	−.021 (−2.23)	−.010 (−2.07)	−.004 (−0.76)	.002 (0.40)	−.0008 (−0.14)	−.001 (−0.31)	−1.15 (−1.35)	−1.47 (−1.28)	−.822 (−1.25)	−1.09 (−2.13)
F 15–44	.101 (8.45)	.078 (5.90)	.125 (8.63)	.100 (13.3)	.032 (4.04)	.020 (2.29)	.021 (2.42)	.025 (5.07)	−3.45 (−2.70)	−2.01 (−1.18)	−1.78 (−1.79)	−2.54 (−3.30)
FAMSZ	.002 (0.90)	−.002 (−1.03)	−.003 (−1.44)	−.001 (−0.92)	.0005 (0.44)	−.002 (−1.52)	−.001 (−1.01)	−.0008 (−1.15)	−.207 (−1.15)	.347 (1.28)	.095 (0.67)	.061 (0.54)
WORKING	−.054 (−6.86)	−.033 (−3.91)	−.053 (−5.53)	−.047 (−9.53)	−.011 (−2.11)	−.002 (−0.31)	−.006 (−1.07)	−.007 (−2.11)	−2.03 (−2.77)	−1.08 (−1.12)	−1.06 (−1.88)	−1.35 (−3.08)
NOINS	−.018 (−1.86)	−.034 (−3.15)	−.037 (−3.52)	−.030 (−5.02)	−.020 (−3.11)	−.021 (−2.95)	−.020 (−3.18)	−.021 (−5.51)	2.37 (2.33)	3.56 (2.60)	1.02 (1.47)	2.25 (3.84)
FAMINC	−.0001 (−1.99)	.000 (0.04)	.00002 (0.48)	−.00003 (−0.80)	−.00004 (−1.33)	.00005 (1.30)	.0001 (2.44)	.00003 (1.26)	.004 (0.70)	.005 (0.67)	−.001 (−0.21)	.003 (1.02)
GP/MD	−.392 (−3.17)	.002 (1.01)	.017 (0.40)	−.002 (−0.06)	−.081 (−1.71)	−.025 (−0.80)	−.004 (−0.30)	−.021 (−1.96)	10.1 (0.71)	3.47 (0.40)	−.522 (−0.19)	4.01 (1.36)
POPDENS	.003 (0.57)	−.0003 (−0.36)	.004 (1.53)	−.0005 (−1.63)	.0005 (1.58)	−.0003 (−0.55)	.003 (2.00)	−.0003 (−1.36)	.116 (2.44)	−.100 (−0.84)	.131 (0.82)	.069 (2.49)

Table 6.4—continued

Regression Coefficients (t statistics in parentheses)

Independent Variable or Statistic	All Episodes				Surgically Treated Episodes				Average Length of Stay			
	22 Large SMSAs	Other SMSAs	Non-metro Areas	All Areas	22 Large SMSAs	Other SMSAs	Non-metro Areas	All Areas	22 Large SMSAs	Other SMSAs	Non-metro Areas	All Areas
MDFEE	-.010 (-2.49)	.002 (1.03)	-.005 (-0.21)	-.005 (-0.37)	-.007 (-3.07)	.0000 (0.05)	.0003 (0.17)	-.001 (-1.17)	.009 (0.02)	.691 (2.66)	.016 (0.09)	.247 (1.88)
HOSCOST	.0008 (2.16)	-.000 (-0.02)	-.002 (-0.59)	.00004 (0.26)	.0002 (0.69)	-.0001 (-0.55)	-.000 (-0.02)	.0000 (0.05)	.010 (0.28)	-.069 (-1.76)	-.003 (-0.13)	-.036 (-2.05)
BEDS*	.021 (0.34)	.060 (1.58)	.028 (1.27)	.036 (2.18)	.057 (-1.40)	-.014 (-0.56)	.002 (0.14)	-.005 (-0.50)	4.54 (0.79)	5.74 (1.23)	-.855 (-0.59)	1.57 (1.00)
HBMD*	-.580 (-2.39)	-.578 (-0.33)	-.100 (-0.90)	-.099 (-1.26)	-.047 (-0.30)	.053 (0.45)	.018 (0.27)	.029 (0.59)	-6.42 (-0.26)	44.8 (2.16)	4.99 (0.65)	8.88 (1.17)
OBMD*	-.761 (-2.82)	-.008 (-0.04)	.044 (0.71)	-.004 (-0.07)	—	—	—	—	-37.5 (-1.43)	-41.9 (-1.73)	-1.68 (-0.45)	-6.42 (-1.39)
SURG/MD or SURG*	-.677 (-2.49)	.115 (0.82)	.046 (0.60)	.029 (0.50)	-.230 (-0.39)	-.042 (-0.10)	.056 (0.42)	.016 (0.14)	19.0 (0.70)	-2.23 (-0.13)	.264 (0.05)	8.53 (1.59)
LOED	.008 (0.90)	.002 (0.19)	.011 (1.79)	.014 (2.47)	.014 (2.16)	.004 (0.60)	.011 (1.79)	.010 (2.67)	.082 (0.80)	.049 (0.04)	-.628 (-0.91)	-.106 (-0.19)
MIDED	.011 (1.15)	.010 (1.13)	.004 (0.70)	.012 (2.25)	.014 (2.52)	.008 (1.53)	.004 (0.70)	.009 (2.70)	-.933 (-1.02)	-.470 (-0.45)	.543 (0.83)	-.216 (0.43)
SMMET				-.0008 (-0.12)				.001 (0.24)				.229 (0.33)
RURAL				.016 (1.64)				.004 (0.55)				-1.64 (-1.75)
Constant	.505 (3.19)	-.008 (-0.09)	.062 (1.20)	.060 (1.58)	.133 (2.98)	.052 (1.65)	.017 (0.80)	.044 (2.75)	1.68 (0.10)	6.09 (0.56)	6.86 (1.96)	3.88 (1.05)
$\bar{R}^2$	.077	.057	.078	.017	.037	.028	.032	.032	.087	.066	.087	.074
n	14887	13018	12760	40665	14887	13018	12760	40665	1369	1244	1352	3965

Fuchs' rates. This is the group of persons in families with incomes below a poverty line. They were deleted from our sample because many of them may have had Medicaid coverage not measured in our data set. One may speculate that availability effects might be concentrated among this group to an extent sufficient to lead to measurement of an overall availability effect. Since members of this group are especially likely to be in families with heads of low education, the possibility is especially likely.

In summary, it appears that there is little evidence of an overall availability effect for hospital episodes, whether surgically treated or not. With the possible exception of the very poor, physician stock is unrelated to patients' use of hospitals, and beds are only weakly related. It does not even appear that surgery is more frequent where surgical specialists are more common.

7   Conclusions and Policy Implications

The major goals of this study were (1) to show how physicians as providers of inputs affect the productivity of other providers in the health sector; (2) to examine the role of the physician as proxy demander for the patient of other inputs into the treatment process, especially those inputs for which the physician himself bears no outlay cost; (3) to indicate whether or how the physician as provider of advice on states of health and on the productivity of care affects the demand for his own and other inputs. In this chapter I will summarize the answers to each of these questions and relate them to issues of public policy.

Physicians as Providers of Inputs

The results in chapter 3 indicate that the level of physician input may have important effects on measured hospital productivity. Put another way, if one does not take differences in physician input into account, hospitals may exhibit relatively large and inexplicable differences in productivity. Since costliness is just the obverse of productivity, it follows that if the level of physician input does vary across hospitals, some of observed variation in hospital costs across such hospitals may in fact reflect the level of physician input.

Hospitals do vary fairly extensively in such measures of cost as cost per case and cost per patient-day. Often the mere magnitude of this variation is used as evidence for the proposition that hospitals are typically inefficient enterprises: if some have low costs, but others high costs, then the high cost hospitals must be behaving in an inefficient way. This is not, of course, all there is to the matter of inefficiency: hospitals could have virtually identical costs, and still be equally inefficient. Nevertheless, many of the mechanisms proposed for incentive reimbursement of hospitals involve comparison of hospital costs, either across hospitals

111

or over time. This implies that "objective" determinants of the level of cost—things which are in some sense not the fault of the hospital, or not properly labelled as inefficiencies—should be adjusted for before the comparisons are made. Traditional candidates for such adjustments are such things as casemix, teaching status, and so on. Some other potential adjustments such as length of stay or service intensity are more questionable. But the implication of the results of chapter 3 is that there is another candidate for inclusion in the first list: the level of physician input, or proxies for it.

If the level of physician input is not controlled for in reimbursement formulas, some potentially severe biases and inefficiencies can be introduced. Hospitals with high levels of physician input will be rewarded, and ones with low levels of physician input punished. If the level of physician input is wholly exogenous and random, in the short run this will simply mean a capricious distribution of largesse. In the longer run, some hospitals, those with large amounts of physician input, may have surplus funds, while those with small amounts will suffer deficits. The latter will presumably go out of business or contract, while the former will expand.

Since I showed that hospitals, on average, use relatively too little physician input, the immediate impact of this development may be beneficial, since output will be concentrated in those hospitals with close to the ideal ratio of physicians to hospital inputs. If, however, the hospitals with too few physicians remain in business, even this beneficial outcome is uncertain. Some physicians will be likely to leave such hospitals, making the ratios even worse than before. Eventually some output may be produced at lower cost than before, but other output may be produced at higher cost. What is relevant, of course, is not average cost, but marginal cost.

The primary difficulty, however, is that there is no reason to expect this process to stop once the ideal ratio is approximated. Instead, it will continue up to the maximum technological limit of substitution of physician input for other hospital input. In effect, by transferring costs to physicians' inputs (even if physicians are fully reimbursed), a hospital can appear to be efficient, and it will therefore be rewarded and survive. A hospital that cannot or will not transfer costs will shrink or disappear. Since the process only looks at the hospital's cost, not the total cost, there is no reason to expect that it will achieve a solution which minimizes total cost. Indeed, it will be likely to transfer to physicians activities which cost more when performed by physicians in their offices, but which nevertheless lower hospital costs.

In summary, given the caveat about the relationship of marginal and average costs, reimbursement mechanisms based on efficient cost levels rather than actual costs can improve the efficiency of the hospital sector. Because these methods are so powerful, it is important that they be based on the proper measure of costs. One such component which is not included in hospital budgets, but which deserves emphasis, is the level of physician inputs. What is relevant is the *total* cost of hospitalization, including the physician input; this is the cost on which reimbursement should be based if an efficient outcome is to be achieved.

Physicians as Proxy Demanders

The physician serves as a surrogate demander for the patient in choosing the level of inputs to produce health. It is sometimes argued in the literature that under fee-for-service the physician has no incentive to choose the cost minimizing combination of those outputs for which he does not pay directly. Since some of those inputs, such as hospital care or prescription drugs, are a large proportion of total cost, often larger than the doctor's bill, it is argued that such inefficiency can be severe. To avoid it, some method which makes the physician directly liable for the costs of all inputs, such as prepaid group practice, is often suggested.

Most of this analysis is conceptual; what empirical evidence there is is often anecdotal or confounds the measurement of cost minimization for a given level of health or well-being with that of the level of health or well-being achieved. I do not wish add to the store of anecdotes on this subject, but rather show that, at least at the conceptual level, the argument is invalid if the physician is an income maximizer and is free to adjust the price he charges for his own services. In such a case, the physician will not order a high-cost input where a low-cost input would do just as well. For if he were to do so, the amount he could collect for his own services would be less. The physician may *not* act as his patients' agent in choosing the level of health or well-being, but he will act as such an agent in choosing the level of other inputs for a given level of health.

What then of the anecdotes? I offer two possible explanations for the possibility that physicians do not cost minimize. One is that they are not really income maximizers, a proposition for which there is ample empirical evidence. But this is a problem of objective functions, not incentive systems. Indeed, attempts to produce cost-minimizing solutions by fiat will actually be less efficient than permitting physicians to do what they want. If this is the case, there is relatively little that can be done at a policy level.

The second possible reason is that consumers have differential information. They know what going rates are for physicians' services, but they are unaware of differences among physicians with regard to the prices or quantities of other health care inputs they prescribe. Then a physician who substitutes, say, a cheaper but therapeutically equivalent drug for a more expensive one will not find that he can gain from doing so by charging slightly more for his own services. For if he raises his price, even though the total cost to the consumer of his method of treatment is less, he will lose customers.

If this assumption about differential information is correct, the analysis offers a new perspective on the difference between prepaid group practice or health maintenance organizations (HMOs) and fee-for-service. It suggests that one advantage of HMOs, and of competition among HMOs, is that they can make information on the total cost of treatment available to consumers.

Another implication is that current legal proceedings to remove medical ethical bans on advertising would have the largest potential benefit not from the information that could be provided on the prices different physicians charge for their own services, but rather from the information that competing physicians might find it worthwhile to provide on the quantities and prices of other services they typically use. Existing empirical work on the effect of permitting advertising has been confined to a profession (optometry) where the quantity of prescribed services provided by others is small relative to the professional's charge.[1] In medicine, where hospital and prescription drug bills combined far exceed physician charges, both the benefits from permitting advertising and the content of that advertising might be expected to be much different. This is especially likely to be true for hospital-oriented specialties.

A final important implication of the analysis is that if physician fees are fixed, as might occur under various forms of third party reimbursement or under price controls, then much of the incentive to minimize the cost of other inputs is lost. The physician can still attract customers by offering them lower costs for other inputs, but he cannot gain from this increased demand for his own services by raising his price. Only if he were initially in a situation of excess supply, i.e., if he actually gained from producing additional output at the current price, would he have such an incentive. And even here the incentive would be less than would be provided if he could both produce more output *and* get a higher price for it.

Physicians have, in this analysis, an incentive to cost minimize given the net prices of other inputs that they face. This solution will coincide with minimization of social costs only if those net prices are equal to or proportional to social opportunity cost. Even apart from the usual noncompetitive market distortions, I argued in chapter 2 that for one important class of inputs—hospital inputs—additional distortions may be present. The individual physician may perceive the cost of hospital inputs for his patients to be much less than real cost either because of typical hospital insurance coverage or because of the inability of hospitals to price all of their inputs at marginal cost. If physicians do behave in part as the income maximizers described earlier, one would predict that hospitals would provide too much hospital input relative to physician input.

The empirical results in chapter 3 strongly support this proposition. This is in marked contrast to the results found by Reinhardt and others for physician ambulatory practice, in which physicians used relatively too few other inputs.

While these results are consistent with (apparent) cost minimization or income maximization by physicians, they only point in the hypothesized qualitative direction; they do not prove that all of the substitution that would enhance physician incomes has gone on. But they do show that input combinations of other inputs *are* sensitive to relative net prices, as postulated by the theory. There are, of course, other ad hoc explanations possible: physicians may be thought to be overly aware of costs they must pay directly, such as costs of other inputs in their own practices, and less aware of costs they cause their patients to incur elsewhere. Physicians may not be well informed about gross hospital prices. But if hospital insurance coverage is extensive, net hospital prices may not vary enough to make it worthwhile for the physician to become informed. On balance, these ad hoc explanations seem to be more descriptive of the results of a maximization process such as that outlined rather than genuinely competitive alternative models.

The Physician as Provider of Information

The second empirical study attempts to look at the effect of the information physicians provide on demand for physician and other services. With regard to an individual consumer's demand for physicians' own services, the independent variables of interest are the number of physicians per capita, the total or average demand in his market area, and the gross price received by the physician. I argue that information for a given patient is more likely to be distorted in the direction of increasing the quantity demanded at a given price the smaller the average quantity used per capita, the larger the number of physicians per capita, and the higher the gross price. All of these changes are likely to increase the gain by shifting demand. The first two also reduce physician income, which is more likely to lead to a reduced level of accuracy.

The empirical results strongly support two propositions: (1) the availability effects observed for physicians' services come from alterations in accuracy, not from any of the other hypothesized causes, but (2) except for ambulatory care for low education persons in big cities, such effects are of minor importance. For hospital care, the availability effects, while not measured very precisely, and while not of major importance, seem to come from a reduction in ease or speed of obtaining a hospital bed. In particular, the amount of physician demand creation for expensive types of medical care—hospital episodes and surgery—is small or nonexistent. Past empirical work which has suggested important demand creation effects for these services failed to account adequately for the health status of the patient or for differences in effects across types of geographic areas.

There *is*, then, an availability effect; physicians can affect consumer demand by what they tell consumers. And the effect is strongest precisely among those groups of consumers, those with little education or information, for which one would expect it to be strongest. Overall, however, the practical consequence of the availability effect is quite small. In particular, where patients are more easily able to exchange information about diagnostic accuracy, as perhaps in rural areas, little availability effect can be detected. Either physicians do not generally manipulate information in an effective way or, if they do, they do so to approximately the same extent regardless of how many of them there are in an area, and regardless of how busy they are.

The most obvious policy implication of the alternative theories of the availability effect is implicit in what has already been said: if different theories imply differential effects on different population groups, then concern for the appropriateness of use can be directed to those groups most likely to be affected. In the simplest case, where a policy decision about what is regarded as appropriate use has already been made, the theories have different implications about the kinds of people whose use is likely to be affected by availability. Under one theory, availability will affect most strongly those people with what physicians regard as undeserving conditions (whether because they are trivial or because they are uninteresting); under another, it would be those with higher opportunity cost of time; under still another, those with least information or experience. The confirmation of the information-manipulation theory provides suggestions for the design of corrective measures. For instance, the results in chapter 5 suggest that direct programs to determine the appropriateness of use, such as PSROs, would be most useful for those persons whose use might most be expected to be affected by availability—persons in high producer price areas, persons who are less well educated, and persons with chronic conditions. Of perhaps equal importance is the suggestion in the information manipulation theory that estimates of the partial effect of price on use may be biased downward unless the accuracy of information is controlled for. This qualification is most relevant when insurance coverage is sufficiently low that prices received by producers are approximately equal to prices paid by consumers, as in the case of ambulatory care. The policy implications of changing user prices, e.g., by reducing insurance coverage, while leaving producer prices constant, are also important. The intent of an increase in user price to reduce use and cost may be frustrated if physicians manipulate information to counteract the effect of reduced use on their own incomes.

Where appropriateness of use has not been determined a priori, and where the changes in resource availability are to be evaluated in terms of their effect on use, analysis becomes more complex. The value of use of medical care to the receiver is measured, at the margin, by the price he would be willing to pay if he were appropriately informed.[2] In the case in which time prices are altered by changes in physician availability, a measure of the time price would provide an estimate of the value of additional use, if any exists. But in the excess demand or information manipulation cases, results are not as clear-cut. In the excess demand case, we know that the value of use is at least as great as the price, but that is all. But in the case of information manipulation, even this benchmark is gone. Where manipulation is present, all of the presumptions about the desirability of market results is lost. This makes it especially important to circumscribe those areas: the results in chapters 5 and 6 suggest that they are much more limited than is often suggested.

Finally, if it continues to be confirmed for certain parts of the population, the information manipulation theory can suggest a tool for public policy which has not been much used up to the present: the provision, at public expense, of accurate information to these population groups. This information would have two possible forms, not only more accurate information about the usefulness or, equally, the uselessness of kinds of care physicians suggest, from hypertension therapy to tonsillectomies and hysterectomies, but also information on the accuracy of advice of particular physicians. PSROs should generate this kind of information in any case; it might, however, be most effectively utilized if communicated to consumers. Here again, the kind of information to be collected, the kinds of consumers to whom it should be provided, and the geographic areas of most concern could be determined by empirical analysis.

Economic Models of Physician Behavior

The most general message of this set of studies is that we should not be too quick to depart from standard maximizing economic models in attempting to explain behavior in the medical care industry. Supposedly anomalous features of that industry sometimes vanish when more appropriate sets of data are used, while other apparent institutional differences require only redefinitions of price, ownership-entrepreneurship, and markets to make models analogous to the traditional ones applicable.

This is not to deny that there are not some peculiar features of this industry, nor that expansion of producer and consumer utility functions may be necessary in order to explain behavior. But it does suggest that adaptations of standard economic models may be the most fruitful way of approaching these problems.

Appendix

Table 1	Means and Standard Deviations of Variables by Education of Head and Location: Full Sample (Standard Deviation in Parentheses)					
	22 Largest SMSAs		Other SMSAs		Nonmetro-politan Areas	
Variable	Low Head Education	High Head Education	Low Head Education	High Head Education	Low Head Education	High Head Education
RAD	.641	.523	.605	.389	.589	.370
	(2.42)	(1.95)	(2.283)	(1.643)	(2.287)	(1.639)
CONDS	.579	.603	.590	.587	.645	.585
	(.901)	(.831)	(.897)	(.798)	(.946)	(.848)
AGE LT 15	.239	.312	.254	.330	.258	.333
	(.427)	(.463)	(.436)	(.470)	(.437)	(.471)
AGE 45–64	.278	.173	.270	.164	.268	.166
	(.448)	(.377)	(.444)	(.370)	(.443)	(.372)
AGE 65+	.121	.050	.104	.052	.111	.054
	(.326)	(.217)	(.306)	(.223)	(.314)	(.226)
SEX	.520	.502	.516	.507	.499	.518
	(.500)	(.500)	(.499)	(.500)	(.500)	(.499)
F 15–44	.188	.245	.197	.235	.183	.235
	(.391)	(.430)	(.398)	(.424)	(.387)	(.424)
FAMSZ	.382	3.89	4.08	4.08	4.06	4.02
	(2.10)	(2.01)	(2.112)	(1.945)	(2.162)	(1.869)
WORKING	.422	.409	.413	.398	.419	.394
	(.494)	(.492)	(.492)	(.489)	(.493)	(.489)
NOINS	.177	.081	.184	——	.225	——
	(.382)	(.272)	(.388)	——	(.417)	——
FAMINC	99.8	172.3	97.4	163.5	86.8	146.4
(in 100's)	(50.3)	(75.7)	(48.7)	(73.3)	43.0	(71.8)
GP/MD	.234	.230	.255	.257	.535	.469
	(.061)	(.062)	(.099)	(.095)	(.236)	(.225)
SURG/MD	.302	.301	.339	.329	.241	.264
	(.028)	(.024)	(.048)	(.048)	(1.21)	(.110)

Table 1—*continued*

Variable	22 Largest SMSAs		Other SMSAs		Nonmetro-politan Areas	
	Low Head Education	High Head Education	Low Head Education	High Head Education	Low Head Education	High Head Education
POPDENS	23.0	21.3	5.29	5.38	1.06	1.15
	(13.4)	(12.9)	(4.03)	(4.35)	1.74	1.69
MDFEE	10.92	10.98	8.93	8.96	7.34	7.53
	(2.05)	(1.98)	(1.59)	(1.70)	(1.56)	(2.17)
HOSCOST	100.	102.	72.64	75.72	48.49	51.44
	(11.92)	(11.71)	(12.90)	(13.96)	(12.17)	(14.16)
BEDS*	.438	.427	.449	.445	.372	.400
	(.071)	(.071)	(.107)	(.097)	(.196)	(.229)
HBMD*	.057	.055	.031	.034	.011	.015
	(.018)	(.018)	(.030)	(.030)	(.037)	(.048)
OBMD*	.117	.118	.106	.113	.065	.085
	(.018)	(.017)	(.026)	(.027)	(.046)	(.088)
Hosp. Episodes	.117	.098	.098	.095	.117	.102
	(.388)	(.352)	(.297)	(.293)	(.321)	(.303)
Surg. Treat. Eps.	.055	.040	.051	.048	.054	.050
	(.250)	(.200)	(.220)	(.214)	(.225)	(.218)
Doctor Vis.	3.935	4.022	3.131	3.711	3.384	3.496
	(8.221)	(7.041)	(5.427)	(8.478)	(7.882)	(6.650)
n*[1]	4985	2683	3811	3942	4639	3155

1. A slightly larger set of observations was used in doctor visit regressions; see chapter 6.

Table 2   Means and Standard Deviations of Variables by Education of
Head and Location: Persons with Some Doctor Visits
(Standard Deviation in Parentheses)

Variable	22 Largest SMSAs		Other SMSAs		Nonmetro-politan Areas	
	Low Head Education	High Head Education	Low Head Education	High Head Education	Low Head Education	High Head Education
RAD	.851	.615	.799	.434	.791	.441
	(2.81)	(2.12)	(2.64)	(1.79)	(2.64)	(1.80)
CONDS	.722	.675	.75	.655	.813	.658
	(.969)	(.869)	(.983)	(.832)	(1.02)	(.885)
AGE 15	.239	.333	.244	.344	.252	.341
	(.426)	(.476)	(.431)	(.475)	(.433)	(.474)
AGE 45–64	.279	.160	.277	.148	.274	.164
	(.448)	(.367)	(.439)	(.355)	(.442)	(.370)
AGE 65+	.126	.050	.11	.052	.115	.053
	(.332)	(.216)	(.312)	(.221)	(.315)	(.223)
SEX	.540	.523	.534	.524	.529	.537
	(.499)	(.500)	(.497)	(.499)	(.497)	(.499)
F 15–44	.198	.261	.204	.252	.201	.252
	(.400)	(.439)	(.403)	(.434)	(.403)	(.434)
FAMSZ	3.72	3.87	3.97	4.06	3.95	3.97
	(2.01)	(1.96)	(2.02)	(1.92)	(2.04)	(1.82)
WORKING	.420	.378	.414	.379	.410	.381
	(.491)	(.485)	(.494)	(.485)	(.486)	(.486)
NOINS	.174	.075	.176	——	.213	——
	(.379)	(.263)	(.381)	——	(.414)	——
FAMINC	99.4	172.4	98.7	163.3	86.7	144.8
	(49.9)	(76.2)	(49.8)	(72.7)	(43.2)	(71.1)
GP/MD	.234	.229	.254	.257	.531	.470
	(.062)	(.056)	(.097)	(.096)	(.242)	(.226)
SURG/MD	.302	.301	.339	.328	.243	.265
	(.028)	(.023)	(.047)	(.048)	(.121)	(.110)
POPDENS	23.1	21.3	5.37	5.39	1.10	1.14
	(13.5)	(13.0)	(4.17)	(4.38)	(1.83)	(1.68)
MDFEE	10.92	11.00	8.91	8.92	7.36	7.53
	(2.06)	(1.97)	(1.59)	(1.70)	(1.58)	(2.18)
HOSCOST	100.1	102.3	72.78	75.81	48.82	51.28
	(11.9)	(11.7)	(13.0)	(13.9)	(12.8)	(14.1)
BEDS*	.437	.426	.451	.446	.374	.401
	(.063)	(.070)	(.107)	(.099)	(.199)	(.227)
HBMD*	.056	.055	.031	.035	.011	.015
	(.018)	(.018)	(.031)	(.030)	(.041)	(.048)
OBMD*	.116	.119	.107	.113	.068	.083
	(.018)	(.017)	(.029)	(.028)	(.052)	(.084)
Mean Doctor Visits	5.29	4.64	4.57	4.26	4.59	4.17
	(6.99)	(5.92)	(5.54)	(5.42)	(5.68)	(5.19)
n	3461	2189	2545	3183	3128	2562

Table 3

Means and Standard Deviations of Variables by Education of Head and Location: Persons with Hospital Episodes (Standard Deviation in Parentheses)

Variable	22 Largest SMSAs		Other SMSAs		Nonmetro-politan Areas	
	Low Head Education	High Head Education	Low Head Education	High Head Education	Low Head Education	High Head Education
RAD	2.20	1.70	2.10	1.50	2.052	1.08
	(4.58)	(4.10)	(4.48)	(3.74)	(4.43)	(3.28)
CONDS	1.11	.927	1.13	1.08	1.234	.961
	(1.15)	(1.02)	(1.23)	(1.14)	(1.316)	(1.06)
AGE 15	.121	.165	.141	.202	.123	.192
	(.326)	(.372)	(.354)	(.398)	(.329)	(.393)
AGE 45–64	.310	.128	.293	.169	.346	.213
	(.463)	(.335)	(.459)	(.376)	(.476)	(.413)
AGE 65+	.181	.082	.157	.098	.147	.079
	(.386)	(.276)	(.490)	(.313)	(.355)	(.267)
SEX	.593	.651	.613	.642	.575	.643
	(.492)	(.478)	(.493)	(.484)	(.495)	(.481)
F 15–44	.267	.472	.273	.391	.080	.401
	(.442)	(.500)	(.453)	(.491)	(.449)	(.488)
FAMSZ	3.45	3.77	3.85	3.72	3.790	3.74
	(1.91)	(1.87)	(2.01)	(1.77)	(2.10)	(1.71)
WORKING	.375	.303	.391	.340	.395	.343
	(.485)	(.460)	(.492)	(.478)	(.489)	(.480)
NOINS	.141	.092	.163	——	.193	——
	(.063)	(.031)	(.071)	——	(.086)	——
FAMINC	93.1	167.0	96.2	158.0	87.7	140.0
	(46.3)	(76.8)	(49.3)	(75.1)	(44.6)	(72.0)
GP/MD	.237	.233	.252	.261	.534	.504
	(.065)	(.061)	(.10)	(.09)	(.236)	(.241)
SURG/MD	.302	.311	.343	.328	.242	.251
	(.029)	(.031)	(.059)	(.054)	(.121)	(.123)
POPDENS	21.4	20.4	5.50	5.04	1.179	1.03
	(12.6)	(12.3)	(3.89)	(4.09)	(2.03)	(1.56)
MDFEE	10.57	10.83	8.86	9.04	7.372	7.50
	(1.98)	(1.91)	(1.46)	(1.87)	(1.71)	(2.08)
HOSCOST	99.84	102.16	71.72	75.74	48.57	50.66
	(11.7)	(12.6)	(13.0)	(14.0)	(13.7)	(13.0)
BEDS*	.442	.429	.462	.455	.369	.423
	(.063)	(.076)	(.106)	(.104)	(.185)	(.124)
HBMD*	.055	.054	.031	.032	.010	.011
	(.017)	(.017)	(.032)	(.031)	(.031)	(.051)
OBMD*	.115	.118	.114	.117	.067	.081
	(.019)	(.018)	(.029)	(.028)	(.059)	(.063)
Mean LOS	9.24	7.52	9.27	7.31	6.693	5.78
	(11.3)	(12.4)	(20.6)	(13.5)	(7.37)	(7.49)
n	496	218	——	363	529	295

Notes

1. Physicians as Agents

1. Cf. V. Fuchs, *Who Shall Live?* (New York: Basic Books, 1975), pp. 58–59.
2. American Medical Association, *Profile of Medical Practice, 1975–76 Ed.* (Chicago: American Medical Association, 1976), table 41.
3. U. Reinhardt, *Physician Productivity and the Demand for Health Manpower* (Cambridge: Ballinger Publishing Co., 1975).
4. M. Feldstein, "Econometric Studies of Health Economics," in M. Intriligator and D. Kendrick, eds., *Frontiers of Quantitative Economics II* (Amsterdam: North Holland Publishing Co., 1974).
5. M. V. Pauly, "What Is Unnecessary Surgery?" *Health and Society, The Milbank Memorial Fund Quarterly* 57 (Winter 1979):95–117.
6. D. Smallwood and K. Smith, "Optimal Treatment Decisions, Optimal Fee Schedules, and the Allocation of Medical Resources," unpublished paper, Graduate School of Management, Northwestern University, 1976.
7. Feldstein, "Econometric Studies," suggests that it is easier for the patient to communicate his financial position and tastes to the physician than for the physician to provide the patient with medical information. While there is little empirical information, the communication of patient preferences hardly seems to be an easy task, nor are typical medical encounters so complex that informing the patient would always be undesirable.
8. Fuchs, *Who Shall Live?*
9. Reinhardt, *Physician Productivity.*
10. D. Coate, "The Optimal Employment of Inputs in Fee-for-service, for-profit Health Practices: The Case of Optometrists," *Explorations in Economic Research* 4 (Spring 1977):316–30.

2. Physicians and Hospitals

1. R. Evans, "Behavioural Cost Functions for Hospitals," *Canadian Journal of Economics* 4 (May 1971):190–215.
2. For an analysis of hospital cost inflation based in part on this view, see M. S. Feldstein, *The Rising Cost of Hospital Care* (Washington: Information Resources Press, 1971).
3. J. Newhouse, "The Erosion of the Medical Marketplace," in W. Greenberg, ed., *Competition in the Health Care Sector: Past, Present, and Future* (Washington: Federal Trade Commission, 1978).

4. One additional qualification occurs if the mix of inputs used to treat a given case can be altered by changing the mix of procedures. Suppose the cost-minimizing way of treating a given case is to use a relatively small amount of physician time. Suppose "indemnity" type physician fee insurance pays x dollars for this procedure. Suppose the case can also be treated equally well by another procedure which uses more physician time, but for which the indemnity level is sufficiently high that the physician's net income per hour is greater. Then income-maximizing physicians will use this other procedure. This is a specific illustration of the point made in chapter 4, that when incentive neutrality is lacking, least-cost combinations may not be chosen. Here the distortion in input mix arises not from the insurance coverage per se, but rather from the fee that the insurance pays.

5. M. Olson, *The Logic of Collective Action* (Cambridge, Harvard University Press, 1965); Joseph Newhouse, "The Economics of Group Practice," *Journal of Human Resources* 7 (Summer 1972):37–56.

6. For an attempt to measure this influence, see M. V. Pauly, "The Effect of Medical Staff Characteristics on Hospital Costs," *Journal of Human Resources, Supplement* 13 (1978):77–111.

7. J. Newhouse, "Toward a Theory of Non-profit Institutions: An Economic Model of a Hospital," *American Economic Review* 60 (March 1970):211–26; M. S. Feldstein, "Hospital Cost Inflation: A Study of Nonprofit Price Dynamics," *American Economic Review* 61 (December 1971):853–72.

8. M. S. Feldstein, *Economic Analysis for Health Services Efficiency* (Amsterdam: North Holland Publishing Co., 1967), p. 93.

3. Physician Influence on the Productivity of Hospitals: Empirical Results

1. U. Reinhardt, "A Production Function for Physicians' Services," *Review of Economics and Statistics* 54 (February 1972):55–56.

2. M. Feldstein, *Economic Analysis.*

3. Reinhardt, "A Production Function."

4. V. Fuchs, "Health Services Research Moves Ahead," *Health Services Research* (Fall 1969):242–250.

5. One implication of these results is that increased medical staff will *lower* cost per admission. Cost functions that were actually estimated with this data do indeed show that hospitals in counties with more physicians or with more active medical staff members tend to have lower costs per admission. These results contradict the findings of Davis and Manning, which indicate that, in the hospitals in their data, more medical staff members meant higher costs. (Cf. K. Davis, "The Role of Technology, Demand, and Labor Markets in the Determination of Hospital Costs," in *The Economics of Health and Medical Care*, M. Perlman, ed. [London: MacMillan, 1974], pp. 283–301; W. G. Manning, *Comparative Efficiency in Short-Term General Hospitals*, unpublished Ph.D. thesis, Stanford University, 1975.) They attributed these higher costs to the difficulties of coordinating larger medical staffs. One way to resolve this apparent conflict is to note that the hospitals Davis and Manning looked at were primarily in SMSAs or at least in areas in which physicians might be likely to hold appointments at more than one hospital. In such a situation, larger numbers of staff members might well not mean much more physician time input, but would mean that each physician would bear a smaller share of the costs of his cost-increasing actions. A result which confirms this interpretation can also be found in M. Pauly, "Medical Staff Characteristics." In this study costs were found to increase when the fraction of output for which the average physician is the primary attending physician was smaller. It was also found that costs were significantly higher in hospitals in which a larger fraction of patients had a primary

attending physician who cared for three or fewer patients per month. Moreover, no hospital in this study was the only hospital in the county, and over 80% were in metropolitan areas.

6. Occupancy rates of less than 100% do not necessarily indicate excess capacity, because a hospital faced with demand which is stochastic over short periods of time would want to have some empty beds on average. An ideal occupancy rate for all hospitals of about 80% is sometimes suggested in the literature, and for the isolated rural hospitals in this sample a target of 75% might not be inappropriate.

7. The specification used by Reinhardt was also applied to this set of data. That specification takes logarithms of all inputs which are theoretically needed in positive amounts, but is log-linear and log-quadratic in other inputs. The particular specification used was

$$q = A + \delta_1 \text{ persnl} + \delta_2 \text{ beds} + \delta_3 \text{ nlip} + \beta_1 \text{ GPs} + \beta_2 \text{ SURSPEC}$$
$$+ \beta_3 \text{ MEDSPEC} + \beta_4 \text{ OTHSPEC} + \beta_5 \text{ HOSPBDS} + \delta(\text{MDs})^2$$

where lower case variables represent logarithms.

The results are roughly similar to those in tables 3.4 and 3.5. For example, for the full sample, $\bar{R}^2$ was .869 (vs. .869 in table 3.4) and the marginal admissions product for a G.P. was 38.4 (vs. 31.3) and for a surgical specialist 54.7 (vs. 46.0).

8. Feldstein, *Economic Analysis*, pp. 78–79.

9. The latter interpretation is not, of course, consistent with the single-product Cobb-Douglas form.

10. Fuchs, "Health Services Research."

4. Physician Information and the Consumer's Demand for Care

1. I. Illich, *Medical Nemesis: The Expropriation of Health* (London: Calders & Bagars, 1975).

2. U.S. House of Representatives, *Cost and Quality of Health Care: Unnecessary Surgery*, Subcommittee on Oversight and Investigations, Committee on Interstate and Foreign Commerce. (Washington: U.S. Government Printing Office, 1977).

3. M. Grossman, *The Demand for Health* (New York: Columbia University Press, 1972).

4. To see this, note that when the distribution of $f(g_1)$ takes the degenerate form $(1, 0, 0, \ldots)$, then the conditional and unconditional probabilities in Bayes' formula are equal, and so $f(g_1|g^{\phi_1}) = f(g_1)$. If the distribution of $f(g_1)$ were altered to $(1-\epsilon, \delta_1, \delta_2, \ldots)$, $\Sigma_1 \delta = \epsilon$, and if ϵ were very small, then it follows that the ratio of the conditional and unconditional probabilities could be made virtually equal to one, for any likelihood function.

5. F. Sloan and R. Feldman, "Monopolistic Elements in the Market for Physicians' Services," in W. Greenberg, ed., *Competition in the Health Care Sector*.

6. U. Reinhardt, "Parkinson's Law and the Demand for Physicians' Services," in W. Greenberg, ed., *Competition in the Health Care Sector*.

7. R. Evans, "Supplier-Induced Demand," in M. Perlman, ed., *The Economics of Health and Medical Care* (London: MacMillan, 1974).

8. M. Satterthwaite, "The Effect of Increased Supply on Physician Price: A Theory for the Strange Case of Physicians Services," Center for Health Services and Policy Research, Northwestern University, October, 1977.

9. M. V. Pauly and M. Satterthwaite, "The Effect of Physician Supply on Physician Price," Center for Health Services and Policy Research, Northwestern University, February, 1979.

10. Ibid.

11. If enough consumers are able to detect slight reductions in accuracy, the equilibrium level of accuracy will be "telling the truth"; the cost of reducing accuracy, in the form of loss of customers, will exceed the gain from doing so. Even if the number of physicians then increases, and some persons are less able to detect reductions in accuracy, it may still not pay to reduce accuracy, because the cost of reducing accuracy (even though less) still exceeds the gain from doing so.

12. G. Monsma, "Marginal Revenue and the Demand for Physician's Services" in H. Klarman, ed., *Empirical Studies in Health Economics* (Baltimore: Johns Hopkins Press, 1970).

13. U. Reinhardt has discussed this question in "Reimbursing Non-institutional Providers," in *Controls on Health Care* (Washington: Institute of Medicine, 1975), but he obtains conclusions which differ from those presented here.

14. An incentive system in which money income alone induces the physician to act in *each* patient's interests has been discussed by Ross in the more general context of the "principal-agent" problem. (Cf. S. Ross, "The Economic Theory of Agency: The Principal's Problem," *American Economic Review* 63 (May 1973): 134–39.) But his results seem irrelevant to the empirical situation we are analyzing. He concluded that the class of payoff structures or fee-schedules that maximize the principal's (patient's) utility will be one in which fees depend upon the payoff or outcome. The relevant outcome for physician's services would primarily be health. Actual payments to physicians almost never depend upon the final health outcome achieved. The only exceptions are that (1) if the health outcome is sufficiently low and sufficiently unexpected, then a malpractice action will readjust the fee received, and (2) in prepaid practice, improvements in health do reward the agent insofar as they lead to lower demands for his services. This latter incentive structure is also not ideal, since the agent is rewarded for any action that reduces demand for his services, including death of the patient. Why approximations to Ross's ideal fee schedules have failed to emerge in medical care, as in many other places, is not easy to determine. The reason may be that it is so costly or impossible concerning the outcome, and so easy for the principal to dissimulate about the outcome actually achieved, that such arrangements are not really optimal.

15. On this point, see M. Pauly, "Managing Physicians: Economic Theory," Paper Presented at the Symposium on Hospital Affairs, University of Chicago, Center for Health Administration Studies, June, 1979.

16. Monsma, "Marginal Revenue."

5. The Availability Effect: Empirical Results

1. V. Fuchs, *Who Shall Live?*

2. On this question, see M. Pauly, "What is Unnecessary Surgery?"

3. V. Fuchs and M. Kramer, *Determinants of Expenditures for Physicians Services in the U.S., 1948–68* (Washington: National Center for Health Services Research, 1973).

4. V. Fuchs, "The Supply of Surgeons and the Demand for Surgical Operations," *Journal of Human Resources Supplement* 13 (1978):35–56.

5. J. P. Acton, "Demand for Health Care When Time Prices Vary More than Money Prices," RAND Corporation, May, 1973.

6. C. Phelps and J. Newhouse, "Coinsurance, the Price of Time, and the Demand for Medical Services," *Review of Economics and Statistics* 56 (August 1974): 334–42.

7. If the prices of inputs or the quantity of inputs are fixed below the market-clearing level, then excess demand will occur. Increases in supply will then permit more use if this excess demand becomes manifest. This explanation would seem to be the appropriate one for the "availability effect" observed by Feldstein in his

study of hospital care in the United Kingdom. (Feldstein, *Economic Analysis*). It is certain that there is excess demand for hospital beds in the U.K., and money user price is zero, so that variations in bed supply will be related to use because of variations in the extent of excess demand.

8. M. S. Feldstein, "The Rising Price of Physicians' Services," *Review of Economics and Statistics* 52 (May 1970):121–33.

9. J. Newhouse and F. Sloan, "Physician Pricing: Monopolistic or Competitive: Reply," *Southern Economic Journal* 38 (April 1972):577–80.

10. R. Evans, "Supplier-Induced Demand."

11. Ibid., p. 18.

12. A similar point is made by Sloan and Feldman, "Monopolistic Elements".

13. Evans, "Supplier-Induced Demand," p. 21.

14. Sloan and Feldman, "Monopolistic Elements".

15. For a description of the survey and the data, see National Center for Health Statistics, *Health Survey Procedure: Concepts, Questionnaire Development, and Definitions in the Health Interview Survey*, Vital and Health Statistics, Series L, No. 2, May, 1964, and U.S. National Health Survey, *The Statistical Design of The Health Household-Interview Survey*, Health Statistics, Series A–2, Public Health Service, Washington, D.C., July, 1958.

16. Prices are reported in J. Wooldridge, *The Price of Medical Care as Reflected in a Survey of the 100 Largest SMSA's*, Policy Analysis Series No. 10, Mathematica, Inc., 1975.

17. J. Newhouse and C. Phelps, "New Estimates of the Price and Income Elasticities of Medical Care Services," in R. Rosett, ed., *The Role of Health Insurance in the Health Services Sector*, (New York: National Bureau of Economic Research, 1976). K. Davis and R. Reynolds, "The Impact of Medicare and Medicaid on Access to Medical Care," in Rosett, ed., *Role of Health Insurance*.

18. Newhouse and Phelps, "New Estimates".

19. Although price is endogenous to the market area and is affected by the demand creation efforts of physicians overall, it is probably not strongly affected by the efforts applied to a relatively small fraction of the population (e.g., the uneducated poor).

20. B. Friedman, "On the Rationing of Health Services and Resource Availability," *Journal of Human Resources, Supplement* 13 (1978):57–75.

21. M. Grossman and E. Rand, "Consumer Incentives for Health Services in Chronic Illness," in S. Mushkin, ed., *Consumer Incentives for Health Care* (New York: Prodist., 1974).

22. Such effects have been found in Newhouse and Phelps, "New Estimates," Davis and Reynolds, "Impact of Medicare," J. May, "Utilization of Health Services and the Availability of Resources," in R. Andersen, J. Kravits, and O. Anderson, eds., *Equity in Health Services: Empirical Analyses in Social Policy*, (Cambridge: Ballinger Publishing Co., 1975).

6. Hospital Beds, Hospital-oriented Physicians, and Hospital Use

1. M. S. Feldstein, "Hospital Cost Inflation."

2. J. P. Bunker, "Surgical Manpower," *New England Journal of Medicine* 282 (January 15, 1970):135–44.

3. C. Lewis, "Variations in the Incidence of Surgery," *New England Journal of Medicine* 281 (October 16, 1969):880–84.

4. J. Wennberg and A. Gittelsohn, "Small Area Variations in Health Care Delivery," *Science* 182 (December 14, 1973):1102–8.

5. The set of coefficients does differ across educational groups for the nonmetropolitan areas at the 93% level. But the coefficient on BEDS* is in each case larger

for the high education group, which would appear to be more consistent with a time cost theory than an information manipulation theory.

6. M. Roemer, "Bed Supply and Hospital Utilization: A Natural Experiment," *Hospitals* 35 (November 1, 1961):36–42.

7. C. Lewis, "Variations in the Incidence of Surgery."

8. Fuchs, "The Supply of Surgeons."

7. Conclusions and Policy Implications

1. L. Benham, "The Effects of Advertising on the Price of Eyeglasses," *Journal of Law and Economics* 15 (October 1972):337–52; L. Benham and A. Benham, "Regulating through the Professions: A Perspective on Information Control," *Journal of Law and Economics* 18 (October 1975): 421–47; R. Feldman and J. Begun, "The Effects of Advertising—Lessons from Optometry," *Journal of Human Resources Supplement* 13 (1978):247–62.

2. Pauly, "What Is Unnecessary Surgery?"

Index

Accuracy, physician: choice of, 48–55, 75; consumer estimate of, 56; effects on income, 55; influence on consumers, 43; number of physicians and, 56; physician competition and, 55; profit maximization and, 48–55; value of, 53

Accuracy quotation, 56

Acton, J. P., 70

Advertising, physician, 15, 114

Agency, concept of, 6–7, 113–17

Agent as a monopolist, 7

Aides: monitoring performance of, 13; physician use of, 12, 13

Ambulatory care: availability effect on, 80–90; insurance coverage and, 116; physician provision of, 1; physician time and, 2; price of, 61; substitution for hospitalization, 93

Ambulatory visit rate: availability effect and, 90; general practitioners vs. surgeons, 81

American Medical Association's Distribution of Physicians, 26

Annual Survey of Hospitals (AHA's), 26

Appendectomy, 65

Availability effect: for ambulatory care, 65–67, 70–77, 79–90; based on medical need, 65; differences between urban and rural areas, 71; educational groups and, 81, 90; employment status and, 87; for hospital care, 91–92, 95–96, 98, 106–10, 115; information manipulation and, 97; persons effected by, 116; for physician services, 115; sample division and, 79; target income theory and, 75–77, 84; theoretical explanations of, 67; in urban areas, 85; variables for, 85, 87

Bayes' rule, 46

Blue Shield, 71

Bunker, J. P., 97

Bureau of Labor Statistics, 79

Capitation system, 58–63

Casemix, hospital, 27

Censoring problem, 47–48

Coate, D., 13

Cobb-Douglas Function, 26, 27

Competition among physicians: effects on price, 10; level of accuracy, 53

Competitive market, 7

Consultation, charges for, 63

Consumer: demand for medical care, 44–45; health information, 43, 44; informed vs. ignorant, 47–48; knowledge of medical care, 14; response to physician information, 45

Convalescence, out of hospital, 36, 38

Cost: opportunity, 38; physician, and size principle, 21

Demand creation models, 54–55, 66, 68

Demand curve: effect of information on, 44–47; for individual physicians, 50; for medical care, 5; physician